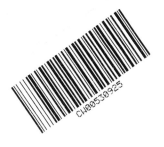

PLAYING L   OR

PART ONE: MEDICAL SCHOOL

JOHN LAWRENCE

INTRODUCTION

Contained herein are my recollections of medical training. I had an atypical story in that I never really planned to go to medical school and when I eventually started, did so with a traumatic head injury. Over the course of this book, and the following ones covering residency training, you will witness the transformative arc as a confused student studying books, goes through the terror of seeing actual patients; to the grunt work faced as interns; and finally the mild confidence discovered as a doctor during residency, with increasing responsibility and experience managing complicated cases, along with the accompanying fear.

While I occasionally lump doctors into clichéd groups, like cardiologists intimidating medical students, don't take all I say to heart. I promise you that while everything I write did happen, the tone of the book is often quite tongue in cheek. I have the utmost respect for the doctors and nurses I worked with; they work harder than most of you will ever know and care deeply about their patients.

I have had many wonderful teachers who encouraged and instructed everyone to work the only way they knew how: do your best; do everything the right way. That is the only acceptable way to practice medicine to them. Thank you for letting me share in your profession. While I occasionally tried to work to the high standard you set, this book will quickly crush any notion that I ever came close.

"The art of medicine consists of amusing the patient while nature cures the disease."

—*Voltaire*

(HOW) SEX CHANGE SURGERY GETS ME INTO MEDICAL SCHOOL

I was accepted to medical school because of sex change surgery. It's that simple. Yes, I passed some tests and jumped through the required hoops, so getting in wasn't completely out of the question. But then, Dr. Doug Ross showed up. That's right, roguishly charming George Clooney staggered into County General's ER, and suddenly everybody wanted to play doctor. As audience temperatures rose, medical school applications skyrocketed. NBC and the stethoscope wielding cast of *ER* had effectively obliterated any chance of my becoming a doctor.

Am I prone to exaggeration? Perhaps, but in 1994 when *ER* first aired, 77,000 applicants, all dreaming of evaluating urinary output shoulder-to-shoulder with Dr. Doug Ross, competed for just over 17,000 available seats in medical school. Unfortunately, that was also the year I applied. When *ER* went off the air, applicant numbers dropped to half that number. So, I'm not joking when I say the only reason the school accepted me—a broke, liberal arts educated, river-rafting guide and flailing environmental entrepreneur—was quite literally due to gender altering surgery.

As *ER* gave mouth-to-mouth resuscitation to medical schools' previously diminished applicant pools, the school selection committees became more discriminating about whom to let in. Medical schools started expecting applicants to pass the required pre-med classes, do well on the MCAT, *and* demonstrate an interest in medicine.

I happily graduated college without achieving a single one of those requirements.

During my undergraduate years at Georgetown University, I studied American Government (I was living in D.C. after all), and English (a language I spoke relatively well), and did not take a single pre-med class. My favorite classes included Acting, Shakespeare in Performance, and a screenwriting elective. I harbored no thoughts of a medical career. In fact, my only exposure to medical school was witnessing a group of swaying drunks holding each other upright while belting out *Sweet Caroline* in *The Tombs,* a popular college bar where I worked. The bartender informed me that this boisterous crew had just graduated medical school. You sensed their chortling and toasting were more than your typical end of school celebration; rather, the backslapping camaraderie and booming laughter befitted a company that had survived some hellacious endeavor together—an endeavor I had no desire to experience.

Early on in college, I had told my career advisor that the only thing I did *not* want to be was a doctor. I was not a fan of sick people, disliked the smell of hospitals (still do), and the idea of lugging massive pre-med textbooks across campus made my back hurt. An answer, however honest, that was unlikely to get me admitted to medical school.

To this day it's troubling to explain why I applied to

medical school if I wasn't really sure I wanted to be a doctor. Why go through the trouble, the cost, and the years it takes to complete medical training? Truthfully, I was a bit uncertain what to do after college. So many careers looked appealing, even medicine looked interesting. Several doctors then advised me, if you can imagine anything else you might want to do with your life, do that, only be a doctor if there's nothing else you want to do. I thought, *well that's stupid, I can imagine lots of things to do*...there were infinite appealing experiences and careers to choose from. And at 21, with life immortal, there was an eternity patiently waiting ahead to do it all. *(Ah, to be immortal again!)*

I did eventually justify to myself that medicine would be a purposeful career; one I could use anywhere in the world; with a possible shift-work schedule that would allow me the freedom to pursue my real dream (making movies) while simultaneously fulfilling some Freudian need to please my parents.

I freely admit a few months of therapy would have been a *far* more efficient means of dealing with my insecurities.

Regardless, my uncertainty later proved to be quite awkward because unsurprisingly, "Why do you want to be a doctor?" is a pretty common question the medical schools ask during the application process.

I want to help people, or, *I've wanted to perform heart surgery since pre-school,* are typical responses.

"I'm not really sure I do," is not what you say to impress the admission committee.

To be fair, I'm not the only person to question their medical career choice. I know more than a few students and residents bumbling down hospital hallways on Saturday nights, missing their family and friends, wondering, *"Do I really want to be a doctor?"* To the frustration of many supervisors, friends and family, I just happen to be very open about questioning my decisions in life.

So how did I actually decide to apply? The answer, oddly, lies in France.

Up to this point I had chosen to pursue a dependable career in law with a focus on environmental issues; however, after a few college summers working in law firms, my legal aspirations dimmed. Nonetheless, after graduating college, I took the LSATs, worked in a corporate New York City law firm, and then, to honor a signed blood pact (which I still have and, yes, drinks might have been involved), went to live off my very meager earnings, credit cards, and occasional payments for illegally guiding skiers through the French Alps. I journeyed with my college friend, Scott, who, far smarter than me, did eventually go to law school, and will appear in multiple hospitals later on.

Trust me, this is leading somewhere medical.

That February, in order to escape the many avalanches crashing down around us in the Chamonix valley, we hitchhiked to visit friends in Italy; during which respite I caught a fever after swimming in the winter sea. When I began coughing up blood-tinged mucous, I decided that a doctor might be more appropriate for my care than my college friends. The aging Italian doctor however, in between huffing and puffing on cigarettes, was coughing up thicker brown mucus than me. I had no desire to catch something more dangerous than what was already infecting my lungs, so I left his office without being seen, which led to a fortuitous meeting.

Back in France, still sick and coughing, I went to the Argentière town clinic and met Dr. Lacoste. He diagnosed me with bronchitis—at least I think he did, my medical French was pretty laughable—and gave me some bottles of pills. We spoke for a few minutes and I found his lifestyle quite intriguing: As I understood it, he treated patients in the morning and skied with his daughter every afternoon. We then discussed *Médecins Sans Frontières* (Doctors Without Borders), the physicians and assistants who volunteer in war-torn regions to care for the sick and injured.

I suddenly became fascinated by the idea that perhaps this was the life I was searching for: living in a mountain ski town; working mornings; skiing in the afternoons; and helping disadvantaged populations the other half of the year.

Now, it's equally possible that given my disastrous French language skills, I completely misunderstood Dr. Lacoste, and what he actually told me was that he despised medicine for taking him away from skiing with his daughter, and that his wife had run off with some feckless fart from *Médecins Sans Frontières*. That very possible translation error does make the reasons for my upcoming career choice appear mildly ridiculous. Well, misinterpreted or not, I decided to go work and travel with *Médecins Sans Frontières*.

But to join *Médecins Sans Frontières*, one needed to be a doctor and I was not. In order to be a doctor, you had to go to medical school, which I had not. I was living on cans of stolen green beans, so the mere idea of paying for medical school was ludicrous, let alone getting in.

Even with my vivid imagination, I knew I would never sneak past a medical school admission committee with that tangential, *doctors without borders* and *tobacco inhaling, sputum spewing, Italian doctor by the sea*, rambling of happenstance. Not to mention several outstanding deficiencies on my medical school application stood firmly in the way—such as not taking a single pre-med class or the required MCAT.

That summer, with medical school dangling like a pipe

dream, I worked as a river rafting guide in the southwest Utah desert where there were no pre-med classes to be found for several hundred miles. There was, however, a required wilderness first aid class for river guides. We spent two afternoons listening to an instructor trying to speak over drunken veteran river runners sharing their favorite stories of injured passengers. No, not much that qualified as a pre-med class. So I moved to San Francisco with a few friends, figuring I'd work during the day to pay for evening pre-med classes.

That first night in the Bay Area, lying on the hardwood floor of our shared apartment, pondering the cost of classes and rent, the time required to study, lack of any cash to buy a bed, and the need to work full-time—my unraveling plan to become a doctor triggered some stress—stress that caused an intense pain first in my back, and then my stomach.

I rapidly deployed my two afternoons of wilderness first-aid river guide knowledge and diagnosed myself with appendicitis or food poisoning (wrong on both counts). Whatever it was, the discomfort clouded my ability to think properly, so I called my mother because her husband was a doctor.

Several months prior, upon hearing that I was considering applying to medical school, he had laughed, told me I couldn't apply, that I wouldn't get in, and that if I did, I couldn't afford to pay for it anyway. I should have listened to him and stayed in the Bay Area right before the dot-com boom struck; I could have made billions, lost everything in the crash, and been happily planting grapes for minimal wage right now instead of still paying off medical school loans twenty years later. Once again, a bit of therapy would have saved me a lot of time and money.

His recommendation was that I go see a doctor. *Well, no kidding, I could have figured out that brilliant bit of medical advice by myself if I wasn't so uncomfortable.* I hung up dissatisfied (mostly because he was probably correct) and decided to go to a hospital. It was 4:30 in the morning. I didn't own a car; Uber didn't exist; and my roommates were at their respective girlfriend's.

I sheepishly telephoned Joslin (Scott's girlfriend) feeling every bit the pathetic friend interrupting their sleepover by getting appendicitis. By now the ache was so intense, I was praying it was my appendix, and not just bad gas, which would have been really hard to live down. Fortunately, the two of them were gracious enough to rush over and take me to the hospital.

When we arrived at the hospital a team of doctors, residents, interns, and first-graders (for all I cared), rushed to push on my stomach and ask questions relevant to my dire situation. I begged the doctors to quickly knock me out, or shoot me, whichever was more convenient for them. Instead, I was sent to get a urine sample; and when I returned, proudly displaying my cup of dark yellow liquid, noticed something was amiss.

All my new caring friends had dispersed. My mother was on the phone and had requested I go to a different hospital where her, *you'll-never-get-into-medical-school* husband knew the Chair of Staff, or Chief of Strep, or some guy that had donated money —I didn't care, I couldn't think strait, I was in pain, and I didn't want to leave the safe environment of compassionate people in this hospital to go somewhere else.

I lost that argument.

Minutes later I was painfully waddling down a city sidewalk in an ass-exposing hospital gown holding my cup of urine. Welcome to San Francisco.

As Joslin and Scott drove me to the next hospital, the pain intensified to the point that I was trying to rip the seatbelts out of the car in agony and then... relief.

A nasty bugger of a kidney stone had completed the painful journey to my bladder. By the time we arrived in the ER waiting room, I was relatively pain-free. I eventually fell asleep on an X-ray table, only to be woken by a cute technician rubbing warm jelly over my abdomen for an ultrasound. She told me that kidney stones were supposed to be as painful as childbirth. Here was a woman being nice to me—things were looking up in the Bay Area.

After that wonderful jelly rubdown, I was left alone in an exam room until I eventually met the ER physician in charge. She was a super-friendly woman who once upon a time had been a fashion model, and before that, a diamond hunter in Africa. After those exotic adventures, she became an ER doctor, and now informed me it was time to perform a rectal exam—and proceeded to do so. Welcome, again, to San Francisco.

The episode served as a reality check: If I continued living, working, and studying in San Francisco—a triad that gave me kidney stones—it would take several years for me to complete pre-med studies. The time and cost were prohibitive, and my only brushes with medicine were likely to be stress-induced illnesses. I pushed down my ego and asked my mom if I could move back home to New York and attend a nearby SUNY school and community college for my pre-med classes.

Meanwhile, Scott stayed in San Francisco where he was eventually arrested for bungee jumping off the Golden Gate Bridge. Not really a surprise however, it was not the first time that Scott's joie de vivre had attracted Johnny Law. When we lived in Chamonix, the Gendarme had arrested him for disturbing the peace, dropped him off in Italy, and told not to come back to France for several days.[1] With all that firsthand legal experience, it's no surprise that Scott went to law school. While I, plagued by seaside bronchitis and a kidney stone, tried to get into medical school. Who would you rather party with in Vegas? That's right, Scott.

I will leave the riveting tales of my state school biology, chemistry, organic chemistry and physics classes for a light novella. I passed the classes, took the MCAT, moved to Utah, and applied to medical school.

I had one final school application deficiency to complete— the sticky point about proving one's interest in medicine. Most of the 77,000 other applicants all seemed to have found an extra lifetime to discover DNA sequences, publish groundbreaking research with Nobel Prize candidates, or at the minimum, provide nursing care to an aboriginal tribe for ten years. Not to mention they had all double majored in Micro-Cellular Biology and Organic Chemistry.

During my past few years on the planet I had worked as a paralegal, a ski guide, a river-rafting guide, a bagel baker, a blundering entrepreneur promoting environmental products in Eastern Europe, a ski-store salesperson, and had taken acting classes. I scoured my brain and found no practical way of whipping those experiences into a remotely convincing desire to practice medicine. My only hope of admittance was to slip in under the well rounded "liberal arts education" title for which I had convinced myself there must be one opening.

Medical schools, however, insisted on some hint of interest in medicine. I had never done anything medically related beyond injuring myself and getting a kidney stone. So I applied to volunteer in the University of Utah hospital's ER and discovered that even being an unpaid ER volunteer was a competitive position requiring an interview. Two weeks later though, having beaten out fifty other volunteer candidates (go John!) I was standing in the ER where a nurse handed me a two-sizes-too-small, poorly tailored, baby blue "volunteer" blazer with a nametag announcing that my name was "Sam."

My ER duties involved carrying test tubes to the lab and wheeling patients to the radiology department for X-rays—work that *undeniably* confirms one's interest in medicine.

One ER story is worth mentioning, however, as it was the one medical lesson I learned during my almost seven hours of volunteer work. Around 3 a.m. on my second and final night of volunteer duty, a patient was brought in strapped to a gurney with a host of policeman and medics holding him down as he cursed, bitched, kicked, bit, and invented several truly creative word combinations. Nobody knew what party drinks or drugs he had actually ingested as he swore he had injected and inhaled every recreational drug known to man. *But how trustworthy could this guy really be?*

The ER team needed to know precisely what, beyond spiteful venom, now flooded his veins, so that they could administer the appropriate treatment protocol. Herein lies the rub—they were going to need a urine sample for an accurate assessment of the night's poisons.

A brave nurse attempted to coax him into sharing a urine sample. She returned in tears. Next they asked if I, the new volunteer, wanted to place a Foley? I had just learned that placing a Foley catheter meant inserting a tube into this maniac's penis. I politely declined the enviable role. Unable to proceed, the nurses summoned the coolest people in the hospital—the Air-Med helicopter rescue team.

The helicopter team had a call room attached to the ER where they waited to fly off and save lives. They would saunter into the ER, backlit and moving in slow motion to inspirational 80's glam rock tunes. Men, women, babies, puppies—all stopped to admire this crew and their gorgeous hair blowing in the breeze of some unseen hospital fan, as they chuckled over an inside joke. They looked pretty cool to a volunteer kid in a baby-blue blazer.

An Air-Med flight nurse named Steve—a square-jawed, GQ-cover type who will show up later in these books, as he, too, goes to medical school—was called to help us out. He strolled into the patient's room carrying a plastic cup and a piece of a PVC piping.

The patient flung a barrage of curses at Steve, who patiently waited for him to run out of breath. Then Steve smiled and calmly informed the guy, "Look, you can either pee in this cup or I'm going to stick this big tube in your dick. What do you want?"

Five minutes later the guy had urinated in the cup and was sitting un-restrained in a chair in the middle of the ER apologizing to everyone for his insolent behavior. This was a great lesson that stuck with me: Humor and a calm demeanor is a much better way to handle tough patients than being stressed, frustrated, or threatening.

My volunteer experience lasted two nights. Time enough to demonstrate an interest in medicine? Not really, but my application would only state that I had volunteered in the ER, not the actual length of time (several hours) or what my duties (carrying test-tubes) had entailed. In reality I doubted I would even be granted a medical school interview.

But unexpectedly, I was...

I showed up at the University of Utah Medical School smiling in a jacket and tie. My interviewer was an Asian OB/GYN who smiled back, looked over my application, and chuckled. "Where's this place you did your pre-med classes? Some state school in New York? Never heard of it."

I started to explain that I'd lived at home and worked part-time so I could afford to take the classes.

But he was on a roll and piped up with an impressive level of sarcasm, "Wow, you got A-plusses in your classes? You must be super smart. Come on, what kind of school gives an A-plus? A joke school? You're kidding, right? It's a joke, right?"

But it wasn't. I had stayed up past 2 a.m. studying almost every night for a year knowing I was applying from a sneered-upon state school and needed perfect grades to compete against candidates from top-notch universities. I had taken the same board exams as those candidates. I had studied the same text-books as them with the goal of not getting a single answer wrong on any test that entire year. I did every extra-credit offered. The professors saw my perfect exam grades, added in my extra credit work, and generously gave me an A+. Joke or not.

But before I bumbled out that pathetic explanation, he told me, "You're white, male and not applying from in-state. You're not going to get in."

He let that statement sink in, then added, with a spreading smile, "How does it feel to experience reverse discrimination?"

Not great. I can still hear that conversation years later. Never shared that embarrassment with anyone until now. And to top it off, he was right. I didn't get in.

I was waitlisted.

So, I waited, waited, and waited, and felt further humiliated by the school's eventual rejection. I should have walked away. But my ego was bruised, and sometimes we do stupid things to soothe ourselves, like texting drunk or re-applying to medical school.

Retrospectively, those previously mentioned months of psychotherapy would have been such a good idea on so many levels. But I was not the wise doctor I am now, and rashly applied again to smother my feelings of rejection and shame.

Wasted emotions aside, I accepted that I was not becoming a doctor that year, and moved to Poland with a business I'd started to promote environmentally and economically beneficial infrastructure products—a minor economic blunder quickly surpassed by attending medical school.

When I received my surprise invitation to once again interview for medical school, I was still living in Poland, despite a lack of business experience beyond playing Monopoly. If I could unsuccessfully feign my way in a country where I didn't speak the language, and had no training in what I was doing, then how much more difficult could it be to convince a medical admissions board of their need to help me fulfill my destiny with *Médecins sans Frontières?*

I traveled back to the U.S., borrowed a car, drove to Utah, walked up the same medical school steps, armpits sweating, fingers crossed, fervently praying that a different doctor would interview me than the smiling OB from a year ago...

Wish granted.

My interviewer that morning turned out to be a highly touted, very kind, and *very* elderly surgeon—too elderly, I suspected, to be safely operating on live patients anymore. I think he was some Emeritus school royalty who had been tucked away in a large office several floors and many corridors away from the hospital operating rooms in the hopes that he wouldn't wander inside wielding a scalpel.

For our entire interview he entertained me with stories about his career and, most importantly, how he became the very first surgeon trained to perform sex change operations in Utah.

He talked about sex change surgery for forty minutes and I

never said a *single* word. Finally, he glanced down at my application.

I waited tensely for the humiliating questions about the state school and community college where I had completed my pre-med work in order to receive joke grades...I waited for derogatory questions about why I was wasting time river guiding, or living in Poland, if I wanted to be a doctor...

But instead, shockingly, "Volunteer work? Now *that* demonstrates an obvious dedication to the field of medicine. You're going to make a *fine* doctor." He actually applauded my time in the ER!

A few weeks later I was accepted to the University of Utah School of Medicine.

Thank you gender-altering surgery.

Do not take the above tale or what follows as a roadmap for getting into or surviving medical school. But be inspired that if I made it through, then certainly so can you. And there is no secret, really. You show up. You do the work. You do it well. That's what it takes to be a professional in all aspects of life.

Let's go to medical school...

THE BRIGHT LIGHTS OF MEDICAL SCHOOL

I didn't like the start of medical school. I had a mountain of exams to study for, people laughed at me, and the lights were blinding.

Staring into those lights, the bright lights of higher education, I had expected to feel excitement, mild trepidation, and perhaps a bonding fellowship with my new classmates as we embarked on the journey to becoming doctors. Instead I felt confused, exhausted, a bit nauseated, and the people laughing at me seemed anything but supportive...although, they did appear oddly familiar. I peered out at them through a dim tunnel...

"What's going on?" I asked.

This question elicited slurred, drawling laughter, as though an explosion had recently traumatized my hearing....

Then I noticed I was in a bed....

Something was very amiss.

Why am I in a bed?

"I need to go study," I blurted out.

Everyone laughed again.

Unbeknownst to me, we were on the neurology ward of the University of Utah hospital, and my concerned friends had already heard me ask the same questions over and over for hours.

Eventually, when medical school really did start, I would learn that patients with severe head trauma often repeat themselves; it's called perseverating, and I was mastering it without a single day of medical training.

"What am I doing here?"

"You crashed on your mountain bike and hit your head."

"So what are we doing here?"

"There's some bleeding inside your head."

"Is my bike OK?"

"It's pretty beaten up too."

"So why are we here?"

"You crashed on your bike."

"I have to go study."

"School doesn't start for another four weeks."

"So what are we doing *here*?"

"You crashed on your mountain bike and hit your head."

Is my bike ok?

And so it went.

A fourth-year medical student, future neurosurgeon, spent *his* night picking rocks out of my face, shoulder, elbow, and hip. While *I* spent the night in pain and repeatedly explaining to him that I needed to leave and study for my exams. He patiently responded, many times over, that medical school had not yet started and I needed to stay in the hospital.

The restaurant where I worked later told me I left fourteen identical messages telling them I would probably not make it in for my next shift, as I was being kept in a hospital.

While this might sound mildly entertaining now, I was terrified.

Even in my brain-injured state, I realized I had destroyed my life as I knew it. So many simple activities, such as laughing with friends or taking simple food orders at my restaurant job, now appeared daunting; forget passing school tests. But the real fear was life itself, being human and sharing relationships, all life depends on your brain functioning so you can communicate and think—and I had lost it all in one bike crash.

At the moment that I recall gaining some conscious memory on that hospital floor (I don't have any recollection of the crash, getting to the hospital, or being in the ER), I had no idea if this was my permanent future, trapped inside a shell of my former self, unable to function, with vague memory of a previous life.

When my friends eventually left me alone in my hospital bed, I broke down crying.

One small advantage to being on the neurology floor, beyond having nurses accustomed to dealing with head injured patients calling them six times in a row to ask for a urinal, because they cannot recall the first five times they called, was that I shared the room with an un-conscious patient. My roommate, Lawrence, could not speak or move, thereby granting me absolute control over the television channel selection. He had shot his wife in front of their kids and then shot himself in the head while driving away—but not well enough to complete the task. He lay supine with his scalp stapled back together and everybody hoped he would die.

The neurology team would walk into our shared room and give staccato orders, "Lawrence, can you hear me? Lawrence, open your eyes!"

And since I was using the last name, Lawrence, I thought

they were barking at me. So I opened and closed my eyes, several times, to really impress them.

"Lawrence, move your finger!"

I wagged all my fingers, figuring I was doing really well. Then, for some reason I have yet to fathom, the head doctor thought it educational to teach me how to properly shoot oneself in the head. I recall hazily wondering why he thought I needed this information, but I listened carefully in case there was a quiz the next day.

Instead, the next morning, against medical recommendation, I insisted on leaving the hospital after a repeat CT scan showed no further bleeding in my head. My insurance, which I thought overlapped with my medical school insurance, had actually stopped before the new one kicked in. So I left to save money.

Aristotle wrote that the best physicians would be the ones who had been ill or injured themselves. Perhaps my accident-prone tendencies should have been on the med school application after all.

The day before I started medical school, I went mountain biking again. One might rightfully question this decision given the painful weeks of recovery I had experienced, but I had amnesia and could not remember what I had for breakfast, let alone the painful outcomes of mountain biking.

I promised my friends I would be cautious and joined them for a beautiful five-hour ride through mountains, meadows, and groves of Aspen trees celebrating autumn glory. And I was cautious, walking my bike down anything steep, rocky, or technical. With the cars in sight, I finally let the bike cruise down the perfectly smooth trail to the parking lot, enjoying my last hours before medical school engulfed my life.

And then I found myself floating through the air, upside down, muttering expletives.

I landed hard, ripping clothes and tearing skin as I crunched through rocks and roots, shredding fragile scar tissue off my healing body, before thumping headfirst into a tree.

A random log had shot between my spokes and lodged in my bike's front fork, sending me flying.

Concerned friends raced to the scene as I leapt up, exclaiming, "I'm OK. I'm conscious."

And then I began to feel violently ill.

I was experiencing what is medically called "Second Impact Syndrome." I would later learn that suffering a second head injury, however mild, within weeks of a previous concussion, is very serious—potentially fatal even—due to increased swelling around the brain. I was gaining all sorts of practical medical education without opening a single book.

And so medical school finally started, this time for real, and now with a second concussion. I showed up for my first day of medical school limping, confused, swathed in bloody gauze, armed with a liberal arts education, and to really set myself apart from the over-achieving pack of future doctors, lacking short-term memory.

THE ACTUAL FIRST DAY OF MEDICAL SCHOOL STARTED WITH SOME orientation talks. I sat in the back row of the lecture hall that was to be our home for the next year, covered in bandages and concussed, listening to a steady cheerleading effort from the school staff and physicians.

We were entering a noble profession, we would work hard, we would be blessed with sacred relationships with patients, blah, blah, bloopy-da-blah blah—I fell asleep drooling on the desk. I couldn't stay awake through droning lectures as my head injuries were triggering extreme fatigue.

Between the exhaustion, severe headaches, and becoming physically lost in a town where I had lived for several years, I was becoming concerned about my recovery. Maybe it was the orientation lectures, but the impossible reality of my being able to study and memorize volumes of scientific material, hit me. During a break from the lectures, I followed signs back to the hospital's neurology ward. The neurology doctor assured me that my confusion, lack of memory, and exhaustion were perfectly normal symptoms of head trauma and there was nothing I could do.

So I kept going to medical school.

We were treated to a series of barbeques, discussions, and one very poignant poem written by a man who had donated his corpse to be cut open in our upcoming gross anatomy course. He described the activities in which his soon-to-be dissected body had participated, the sights his eyes had enjoyed, the beauty of the world his body and departed soul had experienced. It's the one bit of those first days that I hazily remember. I think his body had actually been dissected the year before, but they really liked the poem and read it to us anyway.

The second-year medical students provided the most accurate characterization of the year ahead: "Best part of being a second year? Not being a first year." It was a mantra they gleefully repeated to us throughout the entire year.

We caught glimpses of exhausted third- and fourth-year students in the hallways. Despite their fatigued appearance, they were the carrot on the stick: Survive the next two years of classwork and you, too, can parade around in scrubs looking just like a real doctor.

Many of the other first-year students knew each other from years of pre-med classes together. While I attempted to stay awake, they bantered about the upcoming workload, the professors that would terrify us in the upcoming months, and which books were necessary to buy. I was confused, broken (physically and financially), and exhausted. This whole medical adventure was starting to feel like a terrible mistake.

MEDICAL SCHOOL FIRST YEAR

HE'S GIVING ME THE PROSTITUTE'S PUPIL!

The first year of medical school is essentially a caffeine-induced exploration into what vast quantity of minute details you can cram into your head using obscene or innuendo-laced mnemonic devices: *What are the eight carpal bones and their alignment in the wrist?* Answer: **Some Lovers Try Positions That They Can't Handle. S**caphoid, **L**unate, **T**riquetral, **P**isiform, **T**rapezium, **T**rapezoid, **C**apitate, **H**amate.

In turn, the professor's role during the first year was to uncover the several bits of information that you didn't study, and put those on a test.

Unlike the majority of students, however, I had bike-crash induced amnesia and could barely recall my own name, let alone the molecules involved in the seventh step of the Krebs cycle or what an accommodating prostitute had to do with pupillary reactions.

Answer: The "Prostitute's Pupil" *accommodates* but does not *react*; which means it constricts when focusing on a nearby object but does not constrict to light. Medically it's the Argyll Robertson pupil and most likely due to neurosyphilis, hence the bawdy reference.

Medical students are expected to memorize volumes of anatomy, biochemistry, physiology, histology, neuro-anatomy, embryology, genetics, etc. Lectures and lab studies were scheduled Monday through Friday with exams popping up continuously to keep us focused. Weekends and nights were used to study the volumes of material we were expected to memorize and regurgitate.

During those first months I had difficulty concentrating, staying awake, or remembering anything. Which means I have limited memories to share with you and will not waste your time with monotonous details: we listened to lectures, stared into microscopes, studied lecture notes and textbooks, and took exam after exam. That's what we did for the entire first year of medical school.

The industrious students attended class infrequently, opting to spend full days hitting the books in the library—which was interesting, as many of them were also the top students in the class. I chose to attend class, assuming that the lectures would encompass what we needed to know for exams—and they very well might have, but my memory was on vacation and I kept falling asleep in class due to the fatigue of head trauma.

It was a trial for me to stay awake in any class—almost impossible after lunch, which, unfortunately was when Gross Anatomy lectures took place. My anatomy class recollections are mostly blurred visions, when I momentarily lifted my head off the desk, of our 5'5" bald professor wielding his laser pointer like Luke Skywalker fighting with a light saber. There's quite a lot to learn in medicine and you can't learn it all, but I suspect patients anticipate their doctor having a working knowledge of what goes where inside the human body. I was going to face several mountain ranges of information to review over the upcoming years.

One of the most prevalent visions non-hallucinating people associate with medical school is of students eagerly dissecting cadavers in anatomy class. And one day that first year, we were shuffled off to the anatomy lab, a decrepit shack, in the parking lot, filled with dead bodies.

We formed groups of four students and were told to choose a cadaver from the body bags lying on top of the stainless steel tables lining the room. Rumor had it that cutting through fat cadavers was difficult, so the groups all grappled to stand by the thinnest appearing cadaver.

My gross anatomy foursome included two students who were alarmingly fascinated by dissecting the human body. They had wanted to be surgeons since their time in utero. The other two, which included me, had no desire to smell like formalin, the toxic substance used to preserve the corpses, and were all too happy to let the future surgeons wield the scalpels. My great contribution to anatomy class was discovering that scrubbing coffee grinds into your hands eliminated the noxious smell of formalin that was sure to ruin any chances of getting a date.

Over the next months we spent several days a week dissecting our cadavers piece by piece, attempting to identify every muscle, nerve, blood vessel, bone, gland, etc. The future surgeons in my group were among the bright students that never attended lectures. The third member was innately endowed with enough knowledge that he skipped class and studying altogether. I attended class, albeit with my head on my desk and my eyes closed. So between the four of us, we had absolutely no anatomy class lecture knowledge to help us slice into our cadaver.

The synchronized surgery team hacked through dried brown flesh and yellow oozing fat, occasionally announcing, "I think this is a nerve," or holding up a piece of fat and flesh and asking, "You think this is something important?"

Meanwhile, I read the cookbook-style anatomy book, with instructions such as, "Knead the arm until tender before cutting the head of the bicep muscles transversely." Our remaining team member wandered the room, hoping to spy on anatomical discoveries made elsewhere—technically the search results should be somewhat similar.

All semester we cut through arms, legs, abdominal cavities, and heads until the anatomy tables resembled a turkey platter at the end of a Thanksgiving feast.

Along with full days of lectures and labs, cutting bodies, and staring at cells under microscopes, exam days rolled around with ferocious frequency, several per week. Anatomy exams included both a written test followed by a "practical exam," where we had several seconds to identify a variety of tagged anatomical structures on the dissected cadavers throughout the lab.

"Ooh, look honey, rhomboids on sale, table two"

The system did create a hierarchy based on those exam grades—which I didn't yet know about. The top students, aware of the importance of our grades, continued to camp out in the library, diligently studying for the onslaught of exams. I think they realized that there was no point in learning the actual lecture material. All that mattered was achieving the highest exam score—which did not reflect the copious amount of lecture notes. We could eventually learn how to be doctors on clinical rotations during our third and fourth years.

My routine differed from the top students living in the library; I headed home and went for a run knowing that studying was futile, as my addled brain could only retain information for short time periods. Without any guidance I had started my own brain recovery program. I played chess against myself. I started eating fish occasionally. I continued exercising, which I figured was good for the brain. I tried stimulating my brain while I ran: Count up to one hundred by twos in Spanish, back down by threes in French, up by fours in Spanish, etc.

Late at night I brewed pots of coffee and stared at pages of information until I fell asleep at my desk. To give you an idea of how severely the head injury affected me during those first months, I would often read a page in the textbook, turn the page and have no idea what I'd read, not even able to recall what subject I was reading. I'd turn the page back, and re-read the same page four or five times. While reading, I listened to Bach or Mozart pieces over and over in hopes that if I thought of the music during the exam, it would trigger some neurons to help me remember answers.

It didn't.

On our first anatomy exam I shattered the famous rule of not changing your first intuitive answer. I changed every single answer at least four times and received the single lowest grade in the class.

I would eventually learn about "Recall" during our Geriatrics lectures. Recall is what allows you to recall something from your brain, a function that naturally declines in many people as they age. We've all had the embarrassing situation when you cannot recall someone's name at a party, someone you know; that's what I felt like, all the time. With everything.

Forgetting friend's names at parties was disconcerting. Forgetting all the anatomy lectures was disastrous.

There's a commonly shared joke in medical school, one I took to heart that semester: *"What do you call the person who graduates last in your medical school class?"*

Doctor.

Upon receiving that kick-to-the-groin lowest-grade bit of reality I decided to level with myself: I had no idea how I was going to survive medical school lacking short-term memory or the energy to stay awake. I needed to tell the medical school about my head injuries and hope they didn't kick me out. The advisors turned out to be quite sympathetic (they did want my tuition after all) and instructed me to see the student counselor.

The student counselor was a very sweet woman whose husband had just died from brain cancer. We discussed relationships and grief—neither of which had much to do with my head injuries or helping me survive school. Interestingly enough, however, a new relationship proved to be the catalyst to my medical school redemption.

I had started spending time with a second-year medical student who was one of the top students in the medical school's history. One day she enlightened me as to what students were actually doing in the library.

They weren't diligently studying textbooks.

They weren't even looking at books or lecture notes.

They were trading old exams and memorizing the answers.

It turns out all our exams were compilations of questions repeated from the years of previous exams. The teachers had no desire to make up new exam questions every year, and not much was changing about the human body's anatomy. So, if you studied several previous exams, you could easily memorize

95% of the questions and answers that would appear on the test.

This breaking news revelation triggered two immediate reactions:

1) I breathed my first easy breath in months. Medical school would now be a cakewalk. All I needed to do was memorize old exams and I'd be a doctor. (Ha!)

2) Apparently every medical student knew about the past exam secret except me. I couldn't believe that not one rat-faced fellow student in the trenches had thought to inform me about the old exams. I needed all the help I could get.

But medical students are a ruthless bunch, as only the top of the class can apply for the most competitive residency programs. So keeping the head-injured bozo down was likely a ploy by my classmates to easily eliminate the low-hanging fruit.

Then again, they probably did tell me, and I had forgotten.

Professors did add a few new questions to each year's exams in order to earn their tenure and allow some genius students a chance to excel and gain admittance to the elite National Medical Society of really smart people destined for competitive residencies, Alpha Omega Alpha (AOA), the national honor society for medical schools. I did not even know such a club existed. Apparently they weren't looking to secretly induct me either.

My big break finally came when my friend, the studious second-year student, gifted me all of her first-year lecture books, notes, and decades worth of old exams.

I had opted to save my meager student loan money for meals and had not purchased any medical textbooks. I now came into an enviable inheritance: each of her syllabi was high-lighted in four colors with her written notes in blue, black, green, and red ink corresponding to lecture notes and textbooks. She had also collected every available exam going back to the dark ages. She compulsively focused on her studies into the wee hours of every night while I could not keep my head up.

But now, armed with volumes of pathologically collected information, I became a great source of interest to everyone in my class who wanted to be privy to my friend's legendary notes and exams. And with years of past tests finally in my clutches, I was going to crush and conquer all the exams, and become head of my class.

So I thought.

I took the first exam for which I had spent the previous night studying old tests and quickly discovered there was little to gain by attempting to memorize old tests when your memory didn't work. I couldn't even remember the answers I had studied. Amnesia was a massive pain in my medical school ass. I was really starting to question what I was even doing in medical school.

At the same time, however, I didn't receive the *lowest* grade in the class. Nobody baked me a cake for landing above the bottom rung, but I didn't leave the classroom and wander the foothills behind school in an existential tailspin—like I had after that first anatomy exam result.

I had proved I could now pass my exams. I might even have relaxed knowing that "passing" was all I needed to do, and that middle-of-the-class was fine, that I'd become a doctor. But I didn't want to just pass and do fine, I wanted to do well, something that was not coming easily to me at all. So I kept trying, and slowly, over the semester, my memory improved.

By the end of the first semester I was regularly scoring in the middle of the class; and by the end of the first year my exam grades were somewhere in the top third. And after months of learning a variety of topics that were considered essential for us, we finished our first year.

My short-term memory and fatigue, while improving, were still present. I was quite aware that while I had been able to pass my exams, the head trauma had prevented me from learning the first year material as well as I wanted, an insecurity that, no matter how hard I worked or how well I did, stayed with me for my entire medical career.

There were several weeks before the second year of medical school started, and my now girlfriend, the top-of-the-class student in the year ahead of me, introduced me to a pediatric orthopedic surgeon who had previously been the national waterskiing champion, and happened to be married to Steve, the flight nurse I had met during my seven critical hours volunteering in the ER. She invited me to join her at the Shriners hospital that summer for a sort of internship in orthopedic surgery.

The "Shrine" is an amazing facility where the orthopedic doctors operate on kids who cannot afford expensive surgeries. I was taught to scrub in and assist (more like watch) surgeries to fix clubfeet, fuse spines, and apply halo frames around legs to stretch bones—which sounded just bananas to me.

Lesson one in surgery: do not show up for early morning spine surgery on an empty stomach. The skin along the length of the spine is flayed open and the bovi, a blazing hot surgical tool, cauterizes all the bleeding vessels amongst the fat. The hot August operating room filled with smoke from the burning fat and blood and I just about passed out.

Lesson two: I learned how to properly suture and tie knots. I was fortunate to have an operating team that not only taught me how to suture, but then let me practice closing (closing the skin after surgery) so that I became very adept at suturing. To this day, one of the few areas where I consider myself not a medical moron is suturing. I've done some pretty good work repairing faces traumatized from impacts with rocks, scaffolding, and golf clubs, for which both I and the patients owe thanks to the orthopedic doctors and nurses at the Shrine.

MEDICAL SCHOOL SECOND YEAR

LET ME CHECK YOUR PLASTIC PROSTATE

We were told second year was great for one reason: it wasn't first year. Which doesn't say very much. After surviving first year, we could feign a sophomoric sense of wisdom, like where to park your car—although I didn't own a car. I still rode my bike; rode it up the hills of Salt Lake City, through the University campus, to the medical school tucked against the foothills. Over the years, my lack of a car had allowed various girlfriends' ex-boyfriends, all of whom seemed to drive huge pickup trucks, to mock me. Never mind them, I was entering my second year of medical school and was going to be a doctor.

The second year of medical school focuses on what people associate with modern western medicine: diagnosing and treating disease. Should "modern" healthcare alter its focus from treating disease to also keeping people healthy in the first place? Good question, I agree wholeheartedly; the change is happening slowly, even in traditional medical schools, but for now I leave that topic to wellness bloggers.

The factor that really started to make me feel like a doctor? The second-year classroom was actually in the hospital. Granted, it was in the basement, down the hall from the laundry rooms and across from the antiquated cafeteria—but it was in the hospital.

Being in the hospital meant we were two hallways and one staircase closer to where real doctors roamed. At any moment a hysterical bystander might burst into our classroom shouting, "Help! We need a doctor! Mr. McNamara is having a heart attack!" But the only thing we were really closer to was the cafeteria's lard-laden menu, and the only medical emergency we were likely to encounter was indigestion.

And now for a tangent: It was quite ironic that hospitals, which we assumed set a standard for health and wellness, were staffed by overweight, sleep-deprived, smoke-inhaling workers. Shift work? Unhealthy. Hospital food? Unhealthy. Smoke inhalation? Unhealthy. Caffeine inhalation? Highly enjoyable.

So there we were, inside the hospital, ready to learn, ready to be doctors, ready to study topics relevant to practicing medicine. During the previous twelve months we had studied cells and theories, and tried to convince ourselves that it was important to understand how the biochemistry of the cells in the eye worked. But few medical students wanted to treat cells and molecules. We wanted to care for people and now started learning about illnesses and medicines, infectious diseases and organ failure, injuries and treatments. And once again we were bombarded with exams, often several a day, because all too soon we would be treating live, heart-pumping (sometimes) patients… which meant we needed to learn how to *examine* real patients outside of textbooks and slide shows. And how do you examine real patients? You take their history and perform a physical exam.

An integral part of second-year studies was learning to perform those "History and Physicals" (H&P's), the cornerstone of Western medical care. What do medical students and residents do during lengthy hospital shifts? They interrogate patients about their medical history, do a physical exam, write several pages documenting the entire occasion, and include a plan for how to treat the patient. Most critically, along with the history, physical, assessment, and plan, was the ability to present that information succinctly, and in an established format to your medical team and attending physician.

At the time I had no idea how important these H&Ps and presentations really were; they seemed like something fun to try that we would eventually be taught how to do properly when it was necessary.

The school should have painted the walls in red ink: Pay attention! This training right now is the ENTIRE FRAMEWORK of practicing medicine.

Here's the thing—it turned out, when we started seeing real patients on the first day of our third year, the doctors and residents expected us to know what we were doing because they were far too busy to teach us anything—despite working in a "teaching" hospital. Evaluating patients and presenting them was almost the whole basis of what we would be doing for the third and fourth years of medical school and all of residency, and for some people, their entire medical career.

But again, I was unaware of this expectation. We'd been stuck inside a classroom and taking exams for the better part of the last year. So to be excused from school to travel to a hospital with a group of friends for the afternoon to practice H&Ps, felt like a field trip with no teacher, instead of a critical part of our medical training.

We were let loose in groups of four to nearby hospitals. My

group was assigned the Veteran's Hospital (VA) where a medical "fellow" (a resident doing specialty training) was to teach us how to correctly perform H&Ps.

There was a tremendous amount to learn: what questions to ask, how to examine a patient, what to write down and in what format. We were relatively uncertain of how to properly perform these H&Ps and looked forward to our supervisor's instruction, again, with all the seriousness one might expect from a field trip of middle school kids with a substitute teacher for the day.

Our supervisor turned out to be a busy cardiology fellow who told us to find a willing patient and do the H&P before reporting to him. That was the extent of our training. *Thank you very much.*

So we ignorant four wandered the VA hallways, peering into random rooms, asking if it would be OK to examine whomever was lying in the bed. The randomness of just talking with a patient on a floor did not add to the sense that we were learning something critical. I expected that if H&Ps were essential to learn, they would've given us some sort of protocol to study for a variety of patients, with all the physical exam and history questions we should know for each case.

Instead, we just looked for patients who happened to be awake and coherent—a rare combination at the VA. Most veterans were elderly, and after days or weeks in their nondescript hospital rooms, were lonely—so most of them were quite willing to talk with four disheveled medical students.

We asked the veteran what we thought were pertinent questions. But since we had no real practical medical knowledge, it was close to guesswork. These sessions turned into something out of the game show, *Family Feud*.

Lined up next to the veteran's bedside we looked at each other to see who would come up with a decent question:

Alex: "So, Mr. Brown, uhhh, did your chest hurt when you had a heart attack?"

Not the typical question a doctor would ask a patient, but to we band of under-instructed brothers, such brilliant interrogation skills elicited cheers:

"Good question, Alex."

"Well played."

Alex (sheepishly): "Thanks." Alex went on to become an orthopedic spine surgeon.

Mr. Brown: "Did I tell you about being shot down?"

Tom: "No, what was that like?"

So we listened to Mr. Brown describe missions we were unsure he really remembered, or had just seen on an episode of *Baa Baa Black Sheep*, but we were successfully talking to a patient; albeit learning nothing about his heart attack or how to perform H&Ps.

While the team asked questions, I began to suspect I was missing something in my medical training. Did these other students actually know what they were doing? Or did they too feel like they were getting away with feigning knowledge? I harbored a serious inferiority complex from the first year head trauma and often wondered how much critical learning I had missed due to my head injury making me forgetful, goofy and tired.

I didn't feel like a doctor who should be talking with patients in their beds. I mostly felt confused and looked forward to our supervisor teaching us the secrets of being a real doctor. And nobody told the patients they were supposed to teach us, either; they were, as I would discover for years to come, no help whatsoever.

Inevitably the entire process turned into the veteran telling us about the missions he had flown, which of us looked like his nephew Frank, and asking if we could smuggle him some beer on our next visit. We gathered our pithy information, listened to Mr. Brown's heart and lungs, pushed on his abdomen, and reported to our medical fellow who was supposed to be supervising and teaching us how to effectively perform this cornerstone of medical practice.

To be fair, the fellows were overworked and probably had no free time to be teaching, anyway. Our cardiology fellow also happened to be from Argentina, and came complete with a thick, semi-intelligible, accent.

Week after week we stood in front of him, presenting our history and physical findings. Week after week he found us to be complete morons. And rather than teaching us how to improve our miserable H&P skills, he lectured us about the heart, and nothing but the heart—which did little to expand our knowledge of how to perform an H&P, how to present the patient properly, or how to examine a single other feature of the human body.

His lectures might very well have been valuable for our knowledge of cardiology had we been able to interpret a modicum of what he spouted. I usually understood the first half of his discussion, as he started drawing simple diagrams on a chalkboard representing the heart and its physiology, but thirty minutes later, with the board looking like a complex version of how to build a nuclear reactor, my eyes were glazed over. I'd given up trying to figure out what the hell he was talking about as the more excited he got, the thicker his accent became. The sessions became worthless. Here's an example of one of our interactions:

We'd enter his office, interrupting his work, to tell him, "We're ready to present the patient."

"Already? *Okays. Let me hear the patient,*" he'd respond in his thick gaucho accent. We'd glance at each other to see who was daring enough to attempt to describe our findings.

"OK, uh, Mr. Jones is a 67-year-old man here for a gall bladder removal—"

"Did all you listens to Mr. Joneses heart?"

"Yes…and he's here for his gall bladder."

"Let's talk about what is happens when the heart is with arritmees."

"Ah-rit-mees?"

"Si, when all the hearts they beat different."

We then listened to a non-intelligible lecture on the heart complete with complicated diagrams to further confuse us, followed by, *"Okay, we see Mr. Joneses."*

We then examined Mr. Jones' heart, unfortunately having learned nothing of how to properly examine the rest of his anatomy—such as his inflamed gallbladder.

The really disheartening part for our instructor, however, seemed to be discovering that we had no idea what subject he had just lectured us about.

"What is we talking about for one hours now?"

"I'm not sure, what?"

"AREET-MEE-AAHS!!"

"Arrhythmias?"

"Si, Arritmias!"

"Oh, well, now that makes sense."

The culmination came towards the end of our time together. The four of us students thought we had done quite well under adverse conditions to learn how to do a passable H&P. We presented our last patient to Carlos del Pampas del Fuego and all went to see the patient together.

The aged veteran patient was complimentary, telling our mentor, "These are going to be some mighty fine doctors."

To which our tango-stepping fellow, without missing a beat, replied in English for once comprehensible, "Oh, I don't know about that."

Fortunately there was further training in how to examine patients outside our Spanish-as- a-Second-Language Cardiac Course.

The other physical exam modules involved hands-on practice. We needed to learn to examine breasts, perform pelvic exams, and palpate prostates—what fun. One evening, we arrived in the hospital prepared to encounter a first-year legend: Bruce.

Bruce was an unkempt homeless man who showed up every year to play pocket keno while second year students lined up to probe past his now toneless sphincter in order to palpate his prostate.

I learned of Bruce when another student described his encounter with this icon of the rectal exam world: Standing in a cramped exam room, the medical student team waited with bated breath for Bruce... the tension mounting as they wondered if he would appear. Then Bruce arrived in style: He strode into the room fully nude, leaned regally up against the wall, raised his arms above his head in a sultry pose with urine dripping from the tip of his penis, and ripped a thunderous fart.

The attending physician had been forced to escort all four students out of the room because they were laughing uncontrollably.

Much to my regret, Bruce was a no-show on my assigned

night—likely having a bigger gig elsewhere. Instead of palpating his infamous prostate, I lined up to palpate eight different plastic replications of prostates in varying degrees of cancerous growth on a tray emblazoned with a big pharmaceutical company name. If I am ever called to examine a large plastic prostate on a tray, I am pretty sure I could tell you what stage of cancer it represents.

Apparently a much higher priority was placed on the physical exam of our future female patients; the breast and pelvic exams were not taught on plastic models. Prostates, like their accompanying gender, were relatively simple to figure out compared to the female anatomy. So instead of feeling plastic breasts, we were instructed how to perform the female exams on live nurses who had generously offered to teach us medical students.

We lined up one by one to palpate a nurse's breast while she instructed us what we were feeling. With great objectivity, we palpated breast tissue, learning how to assess benign normal masses from more concerning ones. I was amazed to discover that breasts had lumps in them, and all the lumps felt the same to me. I might as well have tried asking the breast tissue, "Are you a good lump or a bad lump?" The breast exam however, was a breeze compared to the pressure and confusion of the pelvic exam.

Once more we were herded into lines and waited our turn to screw up performing a pelvic exam. The majority of men in my medical school class seemed to have studied their way right past puberty without regard for the evolving females around them. The pressure of performing a pelvic exam caused several students in front of me to break into a dripping sweat.

Their anxiety was no doubt heightened by rumors we'd heard of male students becoming aroused during the exam. I watched the students in front of me; one by one they nervously shuffled between the nurse's legs, a gloved hand raised to receive a dollop of KY jelly, and then they began to glance around the room, terrified of making eye contact, or actually noticing what their fingers were doing.

I think women agree this is not a comfortable exam to begin with; but enduring an embarrassed medical examiner with trembling fingers and feigned vision loss between their legs, was probably not going to make the experience any more pleasant.

Not that I considered myself adroit between a woman's legs; I was a blundering idiot in the field of women *outside* their legs, never mind the pelvic area, but I stepped up with confidence, ready to learn how to properly perform a pelvic exam. The nurse, lying back with legs spread, gave me orders of where to touch her, where not to touch her (several students had ignorantly rubbed her clitoris despite her demanding they stop), where to place my fingers, what to say and what not to say. My glove was on, lubricating jelly applied, ready to go to third base, and I proceeded to say every single thing I had just been told not to. My confidence shrank...

But finally there I was, fingers successfully inside a nurse's vagina.

The instruction continued: "OK, I want you to palpate my cervix." I felt around her vagina, all of which felt pretty much the same to me.

"This?" I asked.

"No."

I prodded around some more.

"How about this?"

"No!"

I started having flashes of sexual ineptitude as I probed around some more. Like my fellow students before me, I now began sweating, and started to think, *perhaps my fingers are too small to palpate her cervix? What if she laughs at me?*

I guessed again, "This?"

"Yes, that's it. Well done." But before I could celebrate my awesome discovery, Nurse Supine ordered me, "Now, find my ovary."

Are you kidding? I could barely find the most obvious thing in her vagina let alone some obscure tissue hidden away in her abdomen.

But I started prodding around inside her vagina again, she pushed my other hand onto her stomach and said, "There, do you feel that?" I felt some tissue that seemed like every other lump, bump, or tissue I'd touched.

"That?" I asked.

"Yup, you got it."

I moved my fingers around again, uncertain I was feeling anything at all, and asked, *"This?"*

"Very good. That's what you feel for; you'll be right on the ovary every time. Good work." She complimented me.

I had no idea what I had just felt beyond sympathy for women having their annual exams. But I figured I would have time on the OB/GYN rotations in my third year to figure out the female anatomy. To this day, however, despite hundreds of attempts, I have never come close to knowingly palpating another ovary in my life.

With this rapidly accumulating recognition of ignorance, we were approaching the end of the second year. We were soon to be wearing the coveted third-year white coats and scrubs, walking around the hospital, under-slept, confused, and incompetent in our abilities to examine patients properly.

The final second-year experience was the first medical board exam. There were ogres out there called the USMLE,

Steps I, II, and III. These were the infamous board exams that must be passed before you were allowed to travel further along your medical training path. Step I was the most intimidating of the exams, and we were required to pass it at the end of the second year.

The grades on this exam were rumored to be one of the critical measuring sticks residency programs used in selecting which students they would interview. If you did poorly on the boards, you could not even consider applying to competitive residency programs.

The exam itself was a massive recap of the entire first and second years. I did not want to recap it then, nor do I want to do so now—once was enough. I drank a lot of coffee to help me study, and kept drinking right up until being told to pick up my #2 pencil. My only recollection is spending most of the exam needing to relieve my bladder.

I don't recall my grade on the exam, but I passed, moved past second year into third and was allowed to wander the hospital hallways donning a white lab coat, the costume that made us look somewhat like a doctor. I'm not sure what the average failure rate might have been, but only one or two students in my class did not pass GO, did not collect a stethoscope, and needed to repeat their board exams. And I don't think anyone voluntarily dropped out. As for the rest of us, well...patients, be warned: we're coming to care for you.

MEDICAL SCHOOL THIRD YEAR

LISTEN TO THE NURSES (SERIOUSLY)

After two years of fighting to stay awake in lectures, we waved farewell to classroom theory and moved to clinical rotations. Rotations are the framework for the third and fourth years of medical school, and the entire basis for the cheap labor apprenticeship known as Residency. In order to experience the various fields of medicine, third-year medical students play musical chairs between compulsory clinical rotations every four to eight weeks: Internal Medicine, Surgery, OB/GYN, Pediatrics, etc.

Walking onto a new medical service is similar to the stress of walking onto the first day of a new job where you don't know anyone, where to find anything, what is expected, or who to avoid at recess—except every time you start to feel comfortable in your new role, it's time to transfer services and enjoy the new job stress all over again. Furthering the discomfort (which would get easier once you experienced a few services) was the overnight transformation to actually working in the hospital.

One day you were a classroom geek wearing a T-shirt and

flip-flops, the next you dressed like a working adult and stumbled right past the classroom into a den of zealous physicians, over-worked residents, and militant nurses. Those grizzled caretakers shouldered the burden of caring for patients in the hospital and now had the added chore of molding bewildered medical students into doctors worthy of sharing their hallways —and until then, making sure we didn't kill anyone.

I spent third year as a deer in the headlights of the medical locomotive. Terrified, clueless—well, stop right there, those emotions sum it up pretty well; but on the first day add: heart pounding, palms sweating, dry mouth and wishing I could just go home. I arrived at the fourth-floor nurse's station, where I had been told to report for my first morning, hoping there would be some instruction...

Across the country the daily hospital routine starts with students and residents arriving at the hospital early enough to examine their patients. This was the first time that not owning a car became an issue bigger than arriving in class cold and wet from biking in a rainstorm. Most rotations required you to be at the hospital by 6:00 a.m. or earlier. And on a cold, snowy winter morning, riding my bike uphill to the hospital was going to be an issue. There was still no Uber, and no mass transportation at that early hour. Hello student loans.

I had already borrowed money to pay for school, saved money to eat by not buying textbooks, and now needed to ask the school, "Can I sign my name again for a few thousand dollars to buy a car?"

Of course you can! Just sign here to acknowledge how much that loan payback expands over the long run.

"Several million? OK, it's better than riding my bike uphill in the dark through two feet of snow."

Alright, back to the standard hospital morning routine:

Arrive when it's still dark outside to examine all your patients, collect data from their last 24 hours, and write SOAP notes compiling the information into an assessment and plan.

Writing *notes* is a misnomer. Writing *notes* sounds like we were Hallmark elves leaving small cards on the patient's pillows, "*Dear Mr. Lederer, hope your pancreas gets betterer!*"

In reality SOAP notes are small term papers.

S-O-A-P:

<u>S</u>ubjective listing of what the patient answered to your questions.

<u>O</u>bjective list of the patient's vitals, labs, studies, and physical exam.

<u>A</u>ssessment of the patient based on the subjective and objective information.

<u>P</u>lan for the day.

After scribbling volumes of semi-legible soap notes on every patient in your care, you join all the other students and residents for a morning lecture before starting "Rounds."

Rounds are the Socratic teaching method from hell. Medical teams spend hours walking round and round the hospital floors discussing each patient in great detail. After Rounds, the team completes the work that was discussed and then gets busy with their appropriate activity for the day: surgeons perform surgery, obstetricians deliver babies, and internal medicine doctors write more notes.

I had no idea what I was doing on my first day as a third-year student. I think I was absent when they handed out a memo with what to expect or do on your rotations. My insecurities kicked in hard, and not for the last time, I knew I did not belong in this large group of intelligent and hardworking people, all whom appeared to know what they were doing.

I remembered to wear a tie and semi-pressed shirt, and

waited at the nurse's station where I was supposed to meet my "team." Just the talk of different teams was confusing. I kept hearing about *teams* and optimistically wondered if we were going to play some intramural soccer games. Instead I learned a team consists of an attending physician (the boss), a senior resident, the interns who did the daily grunt work and we medical students who attempted to do the same thing but with fewer patients. On call nights your team had a sleepover and admitted new patients to care for until they died or went home. We never played soccer.

There were two other major players outside our team: the nurses (who whimsically change sides) and our worthy opposition, the patients. Students were instructed to stay on the nurse's good side—assuming they had one—and not to kill the patients.

Nurses could make your sentenced time together quite hellish. I'm ancient and lived back in the days of yore and pagers, but even today, nurses laugh recalling their favorite pastime, paging students repeatedly with simple requests or questions while the students tried to work or God forbid, sleep.

The nurses spent more time with the patients than anyone else and could make or break a student or resident by clueing them into a patient's status or possibly withholding information. At the start of each rotation the nurses made it *quite* clear that your job was to not get in their way.

Most importantly, we needed to check with the nurses before we did anything with their patients—especially, as I was told on my first day, with the patient in Room 442. No sooner had I expressed my absolute understanding of this rule, than a resident handed me an armful of gauze and bandages, and assigned me the task of changing the dressings on the very same patient in Room 442.

At first I assumed this assignment was a joke, but I followed my instructions and looked for the nurse to let her know I was going to change the dressings on the patient she had clearly instructed me not to go near.

I wandered around the busy fourth floor, crowded with residents and students rushing to complete the long list of morning tasks, looking for the absent nurse. Instead, I bumped back into my resident, who assigned me a new chore—at which point I had to admit that I had not yet changed the patient's dressings. When I told him I was looking for the nurse, he scoffed (residents might dare to scoff at nurses, they were technically the doctors in charge of the patient, but it was still risky) and told me to get the dressings changed.

I snuck into Room 442 and was relieved to discover that the patient was sedated; I could now attempt a covert dressing change with scant resistance or noise to alert the nurses.

Everything was going well as I started unwrapping the patient's dressings—but then he began to moan. I was terrified a nurse would hear the noises, so I tried calming him, "I'm just changing your bandages, sorry, be done in a second."

But he kept moaning, louder and more intelligibly, "Don't... want...changed... Don't...change."

"Yes, yes you do, you need them changed," I reassured him. This gorked-out-on-sedatives patient obviously had no idea what was good for him.

He seemed to relax, his complaints not quite as loud, "No... Don't...Change..."

"Almost done...there we go, all finished." I said in a peaceful tone, as I unwrapped the last of his gauze bandages.

Unfortunately, my attempts to soothe him made no difference whatsoever once his infected wound was exposed to the air.

Suddenly his heart rate skyrocketed—which was mostly my fault for causing him a lot of pain, but I believe he shoulders some blame for being so irritatingly insistent that he didn't need his bandages changed. Regardless the cause, his heart rate went so high that his vital sign monitor triggered an air raid warning that alerted nurses in several neighboring hospitals.

Why not just turn it off, you ask?

Mostly, I didn't know how; but secondly, I was terrified of unplugging the shrieking contraption for fear of turning off some vital instrument keeping him alive. So the alarm was blaring, the patient was writhing, and I was sweating profusely under a white lab coat whose pockets were filled with seven books, none of which contained any information to help in this situation. I'd been told these books were essential to carry around on this rotation, but they only served to pull my coat uncomfortably off my neck and shoulders.

At that exact moment, with my clinical and sartorial ineptitude on a pedestal, the militant nurse who had specifically forbade me from entering the room marched in with a fleet of cute student nurses. I spun around with the dressings in my hand while the patient and alarm both shrieked hysterically. From the shocked look on the nurses' faces you would have thought they had caught me smothering the patient.

The nurse turned off the alarm and demanded, "What the hell are you doing?"

It was early in the morning, I had no idea what I was doing, and was getting really frustrated with the lack of instruction.

"I-I'm changing his dressings," I stammered, despite the obvious nature of my task.

"Didn't I just tell you not to come in here without telling me?"

I nodded yes and suppressed the urge to say anything that

might further inflame the situation. I could feel the heat and the sweat building up under my collar.

"I already changed them," she informed me, "You're off on the wrong foot. Wrap him up well." The patient, now calmed down in her presence, scowled at me, the meaning of his moans and complaints quite clear.

I fumbled with the gauze in my hands, unsure how to rewrap his wounds.

"Give me that," the nurse snapped as she took the gauze away from me. I turned various shades of scarlet in front of the student nurses and slunk out.

Welcome aboard.

CARDIOLOGY

THE SINGLE WORST PRESENTATION IN
MEDICAL HISTORY

My first clinical rotation as a third-year student was Cardiology, an Internal Medicine subspecialty. If I had been able to understand the cardiac lessons from our Argentinian cardiology fellow last year, I might have been mildly prepared. Instead, I naively anticipated some teaching and coddling on our first rotation. But that is absolutely not how medical school works; you are expected to show up and know what you are doing, regardless of the fact that you have never, ever done this before.

And cardiologists were the worst teachers. Egotistical and brilliant, they lorded their intellectual superiority and years of research over you while, if you ask me, hypocritically being disappointed in you for not knowing as much cardiology as they did—or at least not enough to take care of their patients. (Mind you, I fully admit there is a much stronger argument to be made by cardiologists that medical students in their first months of rotations are the absolute *worst* students to have on your team.

As mentioned, the first order of business every morning was to arrive at the hospital early enough to examine your assigned patients and record their vital signs (heart rate, temperature, blood pressure, etc.)—which sounded like a simple enough task since the vitals were kept in a nursing chart outside the patient's door.

First, let's spice things up by adding a ticking clock. Hospital clocks exist on some enhanced relativity plane. In the mornings, when you have patients to see, hours speed by in minutes. In the evenings, when you're on call for the weekend, minutes creep by in hours. So, tic-tock, tic-tock, limited time to see every patient before it was time for morning rounds...

Next, add the morning's typical stumbling block: the chart was rarely at the patient's door. It could be anywhere. Most likely it was in the nurse's meeting room being updated because in a conspiratorial effort to frustrate students and interns, the nurses had not charted anything overnight and were now filling it out in preparation for their shift change.

If you want to have your head lopped off as a medical student, walk into the nurse's morning report during a shift change and request a chart...request anything for that matter. You could probably walk into their morning report asking if anyone wants a cappuccino and they would slap you about the head.

In the last years, medicine, with sludge-like technical advances, embraced electronic records. Patient information is now immediately available to medical providers on their smart devices, which have also hopefully replaced those bloody awful, ear-piercing, battery-devouring hellish devices called pagers. I now return you to life as a medical student in the dark ages of the 1990s:

If you actually laid hands on your patient's chart, it

frequently lacked the necessary information. Vitals might have been taken, and if so, they *might* have been charted and if so, odds were high that the nurse's handwriting was illegible. What's more, the scribbled figures on the page would not be added up, so you wasted time adding the milliliters of urine, vomit, and diarrhea your patient produced overnight, and compared them with what volume had been put back into them via food, drinks, IV fluids, and medicine. This was what we learned in medicine, how to track down charts, add up scribbles, and write them down again.

Then we saw the patients.

My favorite patients to examine were the ones missing from their rooms. They might be getting a chest X-ray or enjoying a heart catheter, they might have become sick overnight and been transferred to the ICU, they might be dead. Either way, if they weren't in their room, I didn't have to write a note. The reverse also happened (no, not resurrection) and patients improved in the ICU and were selfishly transferred back to my care— meaning I had an additional note to write.

If the patient was present, my role was to interrogate them efficiently because there were more patients to see as the clock ticked towards morning report.

I have often stated that medicine would be easier without the patients. I stand by those words.

We were taught a very precise method of communicating medical information using a specific vocabulary tailored to each patient's medical issues. The problem was that the patients were not trained to answer in the same vernacular.

The attending and residents had concise questions about their patients and expected concise answers in return. For example, if a patient had been admitted with a heart attack, the team wanted to know if that patient had experienced any chest pain overnight. It was my job to uncover that answer; which sounds like a pretty simple task, right?

Ha!

Along with never trusting a Sicilian when death is on the line (*The Princess Bride*), comes this tautology: medical patients are unable to answer yes or no questions. It's a medical mystery. Maybe it's the food, maybe it's the lodging, maybe it's the medications, perhaps someone told them I was lonely, I don't know, but for some elusive time-wasting riddle designed to crimp my sphincter, medical patients chose to meander gaily through a meadow of rambling happenstance rather than politely answering my simple questions.

What could be so hard, you ask? Merely ask the patient, *did you have any chest pain last night*?

And in any other rational walk of life, I would expect an answer like, "No. No I did not, thank you for asking." But we were in a hospital and I swear to you, learning neurosurgery might have been a cakewalk at times compared with getting a simple "yes" or "no" answer from patients.

The interns, who only weeks ago had been medical students themselves, and knew the terror we were experiencing, tried to help by telling us what to ask the patients. The patients however, were no help whatsoever. They were consistently the largest obstacles, along with my own ignorance, in the way of accomplishing our work—which ironically was caring for them in the first place.

Mrs. Dunsworth, my very first patient, was an alert and conscious woman admitted for angina (chest pain). I started asking her the questions I had been told were important: "Mrs. Dunsworth, did you have any chest pain last night?"

"I'll tell you something," she replied, "the nurse last night was just a doll, very sweet."

I was uncertain what relevance the nurse had to my simple chest pain question, but Mrs. Dunsworth kept talking, so I assumed it was going somewhere.

It wasn't.

I finally interrupted, abandoning the tricky chest pain question, "Mrs. Dunsworth, were you short of breath last night?"

After hearing about her recipe for fried tomatoes instead of an answer related to shortness of breath, I realized she was selfishly impeding my medical education. "Mrs. Dunsworth, please, did you have any problems breathing last night, yes or no, please?"

"Well…" she said as she pondered this question and the two potential answers I had just served her on a platter. "I was fine last night…but then I ate some broccoli and it made my stomach burn."

I wanted to break down and shout like Jerry Maguire, "HELP ME, HELP YOU!"

But she carried on, oblivious to the steam rising from my collar, "Now, I don't know if this has anything to do with it, but when I got up to go to the bathroom—"

"Mrs. Dunsworth," I interrupted, "You're not supposed to get out of bed —"

But she continued her story. "I got out of bed and when I came back they had taken my tray, so I called the nurse, and they brought me another tray! Isn't that nice?"

"Delightful. Please, Mrs. Dunsworth, were you short of breath, last night, at all? Any shortness of breath?"

"Oh, I don't think so."

Finally. Relief washed over me and I scribbled down, *Patient denies SOB* (shortness of breath).

Nobody informed me that Mrs. Dunsworth had experienced a respiratory attack at 3 a.m. and that she'd almost been transferred to the ICU. I would learn these interesting bits of information during rounds after I reported how well she was doing.

Teaching point: Ask the patient's nurse about anything relevant that happened overnight; then check the medicine chart very carefully for what medicines had been given to a patient, such as the ones to treat a respiratory problem.

It's worth noting that at that point, I didn't know or remember what most of the medicines were used for, let alone how to read the medicine chart, which was nowhere to be found, anyway. As I would soon learn, it was considered important to know what medicines your patients were receiving. And I agree, knowing a patient's medication list sounds like something a doctor should know. But before you judge, remember, after Mrs. Dunsworth I had several more patients to see, the clock was ticking, I had to write a page long note about each visit and beyond feeling overwhelmed, I really didn't know what I was doing.

Once Mrs. Dunsworth and I finished our game of questions and tangential answers, I began a very brief physical exam: shine light in her eyes, look for the elusive jugular venous point (JVP) on her neck, listen to lungs, listen to heart, listen to belly and push on it, feel legs for swelling and run out of room calling back, "Bye Mrs. Dunsworth."

I repeated this routine with the rest of my assigned patients, abbreviating the exam further with each patient until my final patient visit consisted of saying "Hi," and listening to make sure they had a pulse.

Then I tried to write my notes.

Note writing is essential to patient care. Physicians read the chart notes to learn about a patient's care and to understand your thought process for ordering tests or medicines. Insurance companies and lawyers use the notes for the same purpose, but with different ends.

I ran to morning conference where I figured I could finish writing my notes.

The first instruction in morning conference was to put our notes away and next time, finish writing them before conference began.

Morning conference was the first of many opportunities to be humbled during the day. A resident presented the case of a patient admitted overnight and the rest of the residents, the interns, and the medical students were supposed to work through how to diagnose and treat the patient using that pesky Socratic method. First the medical students, and then the interns were quizzed on what information was needed and why, what tests to order and why, what treatments, etc. Then an attending discussed the case more fully and quizzed us some more. I pretended to be mute for several weeks.

When my mute bluff was called, I resorted to blunt honesty with: "I don't know." I was so intimate with those three words that I became jealous if anyone else used them before me.

But here is the secret to medical training: it's a game of repeats. The common medical stuff happens 95% of the time and medical education was based on seeing those cases enough times to know what to do. For the other 5% of cases you called a specialist. So they asked the same questions 95% of the time and eventually, one day, you blurted out correct answers you had heard ad nauseam for weeks.

And just as you began to feel mild competency on your assigned service, finally able to answer the appropriate questions, it would be time to rotate to a new specialty with a different vocabulary and different questions and you were right back to being a medical clown.

As previously stated, constantly rotating services was the beast of medical education. Working your way through the varying medical specialties in a few short years meant you rotated through services every four to eight weeks. Inevitably it felt like you were only competent on an obstetric service for several hours before it was time to move to general surgery. I suppose the point was to feel challenged, not competent. A point I took to heart for the next twenty-five years.

Morning conference ended and I ran back to the patient floor to grab the nurses' charts with the vitals I did not get earlier, and scribbled my notes as quickly as possible before the steps of the attending physician echoed down the hallway. It was now time to experience the terror of rounding.

As a medical student, rounding was a horrifying, heart accelerating, cortisol inducing, daily exhibit of my morning's incompetence. For the interns it was a tedious process that kept them from their many duties. For the chief resident it was a chance to try and teach the rest of us while impressing the attending with his well-trained team. And for the attending physicians, tolerating the first months of third-year students and interns must have felt like an eternity in Hell, enduring flubbed words and stumbling organization skills along with a complete lack of anything resembling medical knowledge, let alone cardiology.

Along with myself, our team included one other medical student, a friend of mine who enthusiastically embraced what-ever field of medicine we were studying. On the first day of this rotation he decided he wanted to be a cardiologist, an opinion he held tightly until the month ended and he rotated to neurol-ogy, and decided to be a neurologist. Also playing for our team, one intern going into Obstetrics and another intern going into Ophthalmology. With their futures secured in eye care and women's reproductive systems, their goal on the cardiology service was similar to mine: survive. Fortunately we had a very kind and enthusiastic second-year resident who tried to teach us some cardiology.

And finally, leading the team, the attending physician, a Cardiologist curmudgeon who considered all other branches of medicine suitable for idiots. On his good days he replaced his typical look of repugnant disgust with a frozen scowl. My initial patient presentation would quickly rule out any possibility that I might be headed for cardiology.

The purpose of a presentation is to educate the entire team about your patient and to discuss the plan for that patient's medical care: "Mrs. Dunsworth is a 79-year-old woman who presented with the acute onset of chest pain yesterday." You then described her current state of illness, trying to be efficient else your team would strangle you for wasting time. To add to the pressure, you were not supposed to read from your written notes.

"This is hospital day number two for Mrs. Dunsworth, the 79-year-old woman with hypertension and diabetes who presented with crushing sub-sternal chest pain last night, and was diagnosed with three-vessel coronary artery disease by angio. She reports no chest pain or shortness of breath overnight."

You listed off her medications and their doses: "Her vitals were normal and stable (give numbers)." Then you delivered a head-to-toe description of her relevant physical exam findings, detailed any lab results and any studies, such as the X-ray that you had diligently run down to view and interpret in the radiology department.

(On a complete side note related to "running" down to the radiology department, a study was done that measured how far residents or medical students walked during a typical call night in the hospital with trips to the ER, radiology department, the call room, the cafeteria, the various hospital floors, and the ICU —it averaged over twelve miles. So you needed to eat well, drink plenty of fluids, and get sleep because you'd be on call soon. Three impossibilities as a resident however, included eating well, drinking fluids, and sleeping.)

Then you finished the presentation with an assessment and treatment plan: "A 79-year-old woman with three-vessel heart disease. She is to remain on her current medications and is scheduled for bypass surgery likely tomorrow, so she will be NPO (nothing to eat or drink) after midnight."

The attending then quizzed the students and interns on anything pertinent to this patient.

That would have been a decent presentation.

That is how it worked in theory.

Let me now describe my actual initial presentation: Staring at my written notes, heart pounding, sweat pooling, I began to ramble, "Uh, Mrs. Dunsworth…is it Dunsworth or Dunworth? Well, she's a 97-year woman who had chest pain—Sorry, 79-year old—"

"Will you speak up?" interrupted the hard-of-hearing attending.

"Mrs. Dunsword had chest pain and came to the hospital for it… Well, it was really more like one-and-a-half days ago now, but she never had anything like it before, although she also has hypertension as a risk factor but she says she never smoked and last night she said she did well…except the dinner made her blood pressure go up, normally it's 143 systolic and she didn't want to take her medicines—"

"Excuse me," the attending brusquely interrupted my idiotic and useless discord for what I assumed would be a teaching moment. "Just because you are confused, does not mean you have to make the rest of us so."

Ah, constructive criticism for this, the all-time worst presentation in the history of medicine.

That was a lovely comment I never forgot.

"What medications is she on?" the attending asked me, no longer interested in my poor attempt to present the patient. He just wanted to hear her medical facts and to move on.

An increasing stream of sweat ran down my back as I fumbled through my notes, "She takes aspirin every day and is on metoprolol—"

"How much lopressor is she taking?" asked the attending.

Great, I've got a deaf attending. "I said *metoprolol.*"

The resident nudged me, whispering, "Lopressor is metoprolol."

"You have to know your patient's medication list, both trade and generic names," responded the attending as I scrambled through pages of scribbled notes looking for the dosage and realizing that in terms of relativity, I was signed on to the longest month of my life.

The resident rescued me: "She's on 50 BID of lopressor."

"Yeah," I uselessly piped in, "Its 50 of lopressor." By now the interns were finishing their own notes, ignoring my clouded rendition of this woman's fight to live.

I continued, "Well, she did fine overnight, no real problems—"

"Respiratory was called to see her at 3 a.m. for wheezing. She had an X-ray showing new bilateral effusions," corrected the resident.

"Uh... I didn't know that," I said, in a stunning addition to my growing list of useless statements.

"You have to find out what happened to your patient,"

lectured the attending, with no desire to see patients die on the service for the sake of my education. "Otherwise what the hell are you doing here?"

That's a damn fine question, I thought to myself. One more comment I won't forget.

And so it went, stumbling over what to say, missing crucial facts, ignorant to the names of medications, or how to properly examine a patient because, during my second year, I had a hard time deciphering half of what my Spanish-speaking cardiology fellow was saying.

"Her lungs were clear to auscultation," I stated, meaning her lungs sounded clear when I listened to them.

The intern, who also oversaw all my patients and signed all my notes and orders, amended my findings, "She had bilateral rales and I started her on 40 of Lasix after seeing her X-ray."

I had not heard the *rales,* nor seen the X-ray, nor known about the breathing problem overnight, nor anything about the new medication. And to top it off, I was still unclear about all the technical medical jargon regarding what was going to happen to the patient. I knew she had three blood vessels in her heart that were partially blocked, and I knew that the surgeons were going to take over her care. I relayed this information and took a deep breath. My first patient presentation, however awful, was over.

Rather than educating my team about my patient's current medical condition, however, I had instead experienced her health status as a revelation. It would only take a few minutes to get my heart rate under 140.

The attending suddenly asked, "Which vessels are involved?"

The heart vessels, I wanted to say, but flippancy was not my friend at this moment and instead I looked through my notes which I knew perfectly well contained zero information regarding which blood vessels were clogged and responsible for furthering my medical chagrin.

"You have to know these things," continued our disgusted leader. "Why is she having the CABG?" (Coronary-Artery-Bypass-Graft, pronounced, "cabbage")

Because she needs it almost slipped out, but that was probably not the right answer either. So I shrugged my shoulders and my three favorite words, "I don't know" slipped effortlessly from my mouth.

My oblivion allowed the resident to educate us regarding some random heart vessel study: "The Scandinavian UFFDA trial[1] in 1992 proving that three-vessel disease with greater than 80% occlusion of the two greater vessels showed 70% improvement in mortality if CABG was performed over stenting."

I wasn't aware of any such trials and still had no idea which vessels we were even talking about. In fact, at this point I could barely remember where to find Scandinavia on a map, *and come to think of it, why were they studying heart attacks? They all eat muesli cereal and cross-country ski every day. There's no heart disease in Scandinavia. I've seen those Norwegian sweater catalogues and they're all healthy, beautiful people. They should be studying why they are all so healthy and beautiful, not fudging up heart attack studies to make me look stupid. From now on they can be referred to as the Scandinavian Conspiracy Studies because I will never learn them well enough to ramble off their conclusions in rounds. Why not? I didn't have time.*

I could barely see my patients let alone study what countries had chosen to pour money into research designed to highlight my resemblance to the town simpleton. Secondly, I didn't want to. If I heard anything enough times, perhaps it would stick. That philosophy, repetition ad nauseam, was the heart of western medical education and I was embracing it in on my first day.

Suddenly I realized the whole team was in Mrs. Dunsworth's room saying hello and listening to her heart and lungs—those nice clear lungs I had just been informed were full of rales. That was one way of learning that "rales" were the Rice Crispy crackling sounds in her chest signifying that her lungs were filling with fluid. Fluid in lungs is bad. Details, details, details.

I had heard about rales in my second year of medical school, but until I actually heard them, the information was useless. And hearing them after being humiliated in my first of many horrific rounding experiences was a good way of ensuring I never forgot what rales sounded like. Yes indeed, a bit of method to the madness of fear-based teaching.

The rounding would get easier as I learned the protocols and heard other people perform presentations over and over and over. But in those initial days, it sucked.

After rounding on every patient our team was covering, it was off to noon conference, which was the same as morning conference except it was in the afternoon and instead of bagels and doughnuts, they had a drug company-sponsored lunch. For some reason that first month, every drug representative brought us pizza. For one month I lived on bagels, doughnuts, and pizza—healthcare at its finest. Eating pizza and receiving a free pen that said, "DIFLUCAN" was the highlight of my day.

After yet another hour of lecture on such wondrous topics as hypernatremia, hyponatremia, or idiopathic thrombocytopenia, topics never to be mastered, no matter how many times they were revisited over the next years, I started to think about what a better life the drug reps led. They had friendlier hours, less stress, better pay—they were tan and smiling, what the hell was I doing? Before such thoughts triggered a student mutiny, it was back to the patient floor to order drugs and tests for some patients, while sending others home, which required playing social coordinator: organizing transportation, prescriptions, medical care at home, and follow up plans... and then, best of all, finishing those blasted notes with a new pen advertising improved treatment of female yeast infections.

Eventually the day's work was complete and the options were to go home or settle in for the night if you were on-call.

The call night was a grand adventure in sleep deprivation and cafeteria survival. You entered the hospital early that morning, all too aware that you were not leaving the institutional prison, complete with appropriate food, until sometime the following day. And being on-call meant you could exchange your shirt and tie for scrubs because sleepovers meant wearing pajamas.

Scrubs were one of the many issues that formed a rivalry between surgical and medical residents. Medicine residents often wore khaki pants, scrub tops and their stethoscope around their neck. Surgical residents never wore scrubs during the day outside the operating room, nor did they dangle stethoscopes around their necks (Did you know the guy that invented the stethoscope was some French guy named Le Neck? Ok, actually it was Laennec, but close enough.) If a surgical resident had operated all night, she would still shower (maybe) and wear a blouse, skirt, pants, whatever, but not scrubs. And never, ever would you see a surgical resident with scrubs tucked into khaki pants.

So the surgeons thought the medicine people looked ridiculous. But as a student, it looked cool to be in scrubs, you looked like a working doctor instead of a lost medical student. And don't forget, *ER* was still the hot television show and those actors made wearing scrubs look like you were guaranteed to save a life before hitting a bar with your co-workers.

The major difficulty with wearing scrubs on-call was that our team was not given any to wear. Our resident divided the team up so that while he and an intern admitted a patient from the ER to the hospital floor, the other intern, along with we medical students, hunted down scrubs for the team. In terms of games played by teams, the scrub hunt was close to capture the flag. Scrubs were stocked in the OR changing rooms, which required a numerical code for access. We considered waiting outside the OR and running in to filch scrubs when somebody opened the door, but we looked suspicious hiding in the hall-way, and I was afraid a surgical nurse would spot me taking them and beat me up. Surgical nurses are frightening.

The obstetric (OB) people also had scrubs, but their nurses were bigger than the surgical nurses. While the OB nurses appeared slower, and I figured we could take them in a sprint, their scrub lockers had padlocks.

So we moved for option three, the ER, which stocked scrubs and was often a place of chaos and confusion. While the intern distracted the ER nurses, we students grabbed a handful of scrubs and scuttled out to check our booty. Inevitably we obtained ill-fitting sizes and mismatched colors and spent the nights looking like hospital orphans in a Dickens novel, forced to grovel and steal clothes and food.

The on-call night for students was actually quite tame; the resident rarely asked you to admit more than one patient. It was the interns who spent sleepless nights admitting all the new patients while also cruising around the hospital floors taking care of everyone already admitted, ordering labs and X-rays and medicines for everything from headaches and nausea, to blood clots in lungs, and cardiac arrests.

Even though call nights were exhausting, they provided us with the best learning opportunities. Call nights were when we admitted patients and worked through the process of figuring out what was wrong and how to treat them. Along with admitting patients to the hospital, your team was also responsible for any "medicine" floor patients that worsened or had issues overnight. Patients usually got sick or coded at night—it was just one of those rules. So call nights presented the opportunity to rapidly evaluate somebody having chest pain and to decide what to do. I believe this is one reason it is impossible to eliminate call from residency schedules; despite the long hours, they present the best chance to actually practice medicine.

Another practical advantage of being on-call was being in the hospital at an early hour. We woke our sleeping patients so that for once, we could finish our morning work on time. I soon discovered that medicine mostly involved asking patients about their bodily functions. After a few weeks, my relationships with patients were based on conversations such as, "Morning Mrs. Hatch, how many bowel movements did you have yesterday?" Or, "So, Frank, did you vomit last night? Any blood in your bowel movement?" And, "Mr. Geiger, excuse me sir, have you been passing gas? Not yet? Well then, no food for you."

It was a strange existence for me, just imagining that the next years of my life would entail these early morning bowel movement and gas passing conversations; then again, it was so much worse for the patients, lying in shoddy robes, stuck with needles, and pumped with medicines that would make any of us goofy. Then, to top it off, they were forced to answer personal bodily function questions from a medical student.

Fortunately for all of us involved, the rotation eventually ended. I'd be surprised if the attending cardiologists didn't go out and get rip-roaring drunk together for having survived another July with medical students.

I didn't leave that rotation feeling I had learned much about cardiology. If anything I learned the reality that the next years would involve a lot of paperwork, and a lot of catching up on what I had not adequately learned due to my head injuries.

Then again, maybe every student felt that way on initial rotations, a bit stunned and hoping it would eventually get better; which, one day it would.

If you're going through Hell... Keep going – Winston Churchill

OBSTETRICS

THE CIRCLE OF LIFE

Welcome to the labor and delivery deck. Working on the "deck" sounded exciting, like we were shipping off on an aircraft carrier. Back in reality, we were embarking on the Obstetrics (OB) rotation at the University hospital and the deck was where you gathered to monitor the women in labor. There was much to fear about this baby delivering service, one that combined long work hours with attendings, residents, and nurses whose reputations were anything but maternal.

Medical students started their morning by examining all the mothers who had delivered babies; patient notes were to be written before 6:45 a.m. This required us being in the hospital by 5:30 a.m. in order to review charts and wake up all the new mothers to see if they had been able to urinate during the night —which in turn meant that my wakeup alarm went off before 5:00 a.m. every morning. There were plenty of good parking spots at this hour.

Then there was the call schedule. Our student team was

short one person and we were left to cover call every third night. On top of which the aforementioned nurses, residents and attendings had a reputation for leaving medical students in tears.

"That is not acceptable," was our Chief Resident's favorite sentence. We heard it quite frequently.

The obstetric doctors and nurses had scheduled lectures our first two days to teach us how to perform important tasks, like delivering a baby. Apparently there was more to catching a newborn than donning gloves and pulling.

We needed to learn essential skills, like feeling the top of a baby's skull inside the mother to assess which way their head was facing for delivery. We also needed to learn when to treat mothers and babies with antibiotics, how to measure cervical dilation, and most importantly, how not to get on the nurses' bad side.

The nurses ran the show and their rules were simple: 1) Do what they said, and 2) Do nothing without asking them first. If you broke either rule they would kill you—which was not said in jest. By now we were petrified of breathing on the deck without asking. And the most important rule: Do not ever, Ever, *EVER* go into a patient's room without asking a nurse first. The nurses considered themselves elite militant body-guards to new mothers.

Halfway through the first day of lectures I received a phone call that my friend Scott was looking for me, which was abnormal because our daily conversations were never impor-tant enough to leave a message. Our discussions were usually about the weekend's bike ride or how we could get jobs more interesting than being a medical student or a corporate lawyer.

Minutes later I received a page from my girlfriend, the brilliant and top-of-her medical class student with meticulous notes.

I stepped out of the room and called her back.

Before I could say anything on the phone, she told me, "John Schlesinger died in a car accident this morning."

Time stopped. My body went numb. I can forever hear her voice and those words.

Scott and I were very close to John and his family. John was like a younger brother to us both. He had spent most of his last summers living with us and we had shared countless hikes, bike rides and phone calls in deep conversations about life. He burst with wit and humor—the type of guy that could have a room of children and adults all doubled over laughing uncontrollably. He had just graduated with a Master's degree in creative writing from Stanford University, and was moving to Europe to race bicycles and write news articles.

I was later told I walked back into the lecture room looking like I'd seen a ghost. I told nobody about the call. That night several of us flew from Salt Lake City to meet his family in New York as they arrived home from a vacation.

There are no words for the wail of pain from parents who have lost a child. A pain you never want to contemplate and cannot alleviate.

As a third-year medical student, I didn't believe I had any rights whatsoever. So after taking the redeye to New York without sleeping, then staying up the next night as people arrived from around the country to grieve with the family, I flew back to the hospital because I was on call and was expected to be present.

I had barely slept in over sixty hours and had missed the majority of lectures that explained how to do anything medical on the labor and delivery deck.

Derek, the resident in charge that evening, assigned me my first patient for the night. Apparently she was close to delivering her baby.

Sensing that I was a bit overwhelmed, Derek assured me, "We'll start you off with someone easy and straightforward; she's super nice and healthy. She's young and speaks English." Many patients at the university hospital were Spanish-speaking only. "Go introduce yourself so you're not a new face in the room for the delivery."

As I knocked on the door to the patient's room, my lack of sleep fried neurons received a mild jolt of adrenaline as I began thinking how incredible my first real delivery was going to be— despite not really being sure what I was supposed to do. I was about to welcome a new baby into the world.

I opened the door to this nice woman's room and standing there, glaring at me with a demonic stare, was the Tasmanian Devil, pregnant and wearing a MuuMuu.

"WHO THE FUCK ARE YOU?" she hollered.

"I, I...uh, I'm the medical student," I stammered back.

"WHAT THE FUCK ARE YOU DOING HERE?"

"I, uh, I'm going to be here to uh, deliver—"

"GET THE FUCK OUT NOW! NOW, GODDAMNIT, NOW!!!"

I ran out of the room and the door slammed behind me.

I did not deliver her baby. I did not even go near her room again. I began to wonder what good my next weeks would be if fire-breathing dragon mothers all yelled at me and I never delivered a single baby.

Derek explained that my terrifying experience was not normal and usually the patients knew the medical students were there to work and learn. She had been too close to delivery to push the point. As far as I was concerned she was a mean-spirited devil woman unleashed from Hades.

The next morning I started my new morning ritual, visiting all the patients who had delivered the night before. Luck of the draw, I was forced to go see the same shrew beast that had yelled at me. It was 5 a.m. The ungodly hour alone gave her justifiable reason to yell at me again, let alone the fact that she had just survived a heroically draining endeavor. I took a deep breath, girded my loins, tucked my ego away, and quietly opened the door to the expected tempest.

There in bed, holding a newborn baby, sat a radiant angel of a woman who smiled at me as I entered. I checked the room number on the door... It was impossible, but it was she, the possessed devil woman.

"Hi, how are you?" she inquired sweetly.

"You don't remember me, do you?" I asked suspiciously, thinking she wanted to lure me closer for yet another verbal scalding.

"No, did we meet? There were so many people last night. Isn't this amazing?" she replied, smiling down at her cherub-faced and wrinkled baby.

I checked to make sure the door behind me was still open and cautiously approached the bed. She did not transform into a banshee, but smiled at me again, so obviously enthralled with being a new mother.

I quickly asked my postpartum questions. I pushed on her tender abdomen to palpate her uterus, fully expecting her to punch me in the face. I felt her calves to make sure no blood clots were developing and then backed cautiously out of the room to finish rounding on the other new mothers. I suppose that delivering a baby releases a woman from any expectation of normal behavior.

That call night was my third night in a row without sleep. The endorphins wore out, and exhaustion kicked in, at precisely the same moment that the attending OB doctor decided to summon the three of us medical students into his office for a Socratic teaching session.

The Socratic method implied that all the answers were within us, requiring only the proper questions to prompt our memory. I seemed at a marked handicap compared with the other two students.

First of all, they were female and therefore had the distinct advantage of possessing anatomically innate clues to the process of pregnancy, with all the correct answers buried somewhere deep in their pelvises.

Secondly, they had both been present for the lecture series that I had missed.

Lastly, during this old-fashioned, hellacious, on-the-spot oral interrogation, there appeared to be a distinct advantage to staying awake during the question part of the exam.

I'm not sure Dr. Sutherland had ever dealt with a student actually falling asleep as he was asking the student a question. One second I was staring at him, hearing something about the baby's head position and the next thing I knew somebody was calling my name and I had no idea where I was.

Falling asleep in my attending's office was one way to make a piss-poor impression, but in my defense, I was severely under-slept, under a mountain of emotional stress, and his overstuffed lounge chairs were really cozy. But you do not make excuses as a medical student. I did not tell anyone what had just happened to my friend and was in pretty good denial myself. Despite trying, I had yet to even cry about the death of my friend.

In the following weeks, the result of this trauma-induced

defense mechanism was that for the first time as a medical student, I became extremely focused on my work and learning. I took extra call shifts on an already busy schedule. I studied the textbooks between patient cases. The walled-up emotion fueled my medical training as I threw myself into every task whole-heartedly, unable to summon any conscious cathartic grieving. That would take another four months to fester and eventually crash down upon me unexpectedly.

OBSTETRICS PART TWO

MAYBE SHE DOESN'T HAVE A CERVIX?

Newly dedicated to the study of medicine, I now prepared to actually deliver a baby. Here is the normal process for a typical healthy patient delivery without any problems: A slightly pale woman staggers down the hallway, belly held out, breathing rapidly. (Unless she was Polynesian—the majority of Polynesian women walked nonchalantly onto the deck mere minutes before delivering, and exited the hospital almost as quickly, merely needing documentation that the delivery had actually taken place for the purpose of state benefits.) The only person more pale and breathing more rapidly was the guy trying to assist the woman. He looked around expecting people to dash out and help this pregnant woman in a time of panic. Instead, the nurses glanced up casually, annoyed at being interrupted from reading a book, and inquired what the woman needed.

The husband, partner, or friend tried to reply politely, as the situation seemed obvious, "We think she's in labor?"

But to obstetric nurses, companions were not worth looking

at and they waited for the pregnant woman to reply, "I think I'm in labor." As a student, the first time I saw a woman waddle towards the labor and delivery desk gasping through a contraction, I ran out and grabbed a wheelchair to help her. However, nobody else lifted a finger because more than half of the women were sent home, not yet in true labor.

So that was the first major task: determine if a woman was actually in labor, getting close to labor, or tired of being pregnant and just looking for attention. In order to evaluate if a woman was in labor or not, she was brought into an exam room and the dilation of her cervix checked. If the cervix was closed, she was sent home. If her cervix was dilated, the patient would either be checked in or re-checked hours later to determine if there had been any further progress to warrant being admitted for delivery.

Cervical dilation deserves a paragraph unto itself; it was the more common basis for admitting a woman onto the deck for delivery. This elusive little measurement plagued medical students and expectant mothers alike. Supposedly, as a medical student, I had studied anatomy and should therefore have understood some things about the cervix—like where to find it. The first time that I was told to go measure the cervix of a woman lying in bed, I discovered I had lost any knowledge of female anatomy and practically needed a road sign to direct me towards her spread legs.

Secondly, I also developed an ability to stammer, "Uh," without once questioning that I sounded like an ape. In my defense (*how like a guy*) the medical student's initial encounters in the area between a strange woman's legs could be uncomfortable. There were no social standards to fall back upon, no dinners or walks to get to know one another.

Believe me, none of this was erotic or sexual in any way—

but to walk into a room and say, "Hi, my name is John. I'm a medical student and I'm here to measure your cervix," took a little getting used to. Not to mention primal mechanisms were kicking in hard and these women, with increasing maternal protection hormones, smelled fear. If my voice wavered these women shot looks that made me want to turn tail and hide.

Once past the introduction phase, however, we got to know each other intimately in a real hurry. I put on a glove, the nurse covered it in KY jelly and sheets were rolled back for me to proceed. Fingers inside the patient's vagina, I attempted to locate the cervix. The woman did not find this exploration enjoyable at all and let me know with many verbal and non-verbal cues exactly how uncomfortable she was feeling.

I started thinking, *damn, feels like a lot of soft tissue here... I can't find anything...Maybe she doesn't have a cervix? What do I do? I need to think of something to say.* Finally, I found something that felt like it might be a cervix. *Good God, she's almost there!*

I removed my fingers and announced the good news: "You're six centimeters dilated. We'll get you admitted to deliver your baby." The patient was so happy to not be going home that she started to give me a hug.

Snap! The nurse slipped on a glove, "Let me double check." She quickly repeated the exam while the patient and I smiled at each other.

Two seconds later the nurse crushed our little moment along with my ego. "Your cervix is closed, not in labor," she said. "Maybe tomorrow." This statement magically erased the pregnant woman's smile and I realized there would be no hugs today. My own smile quickly evaporated as the woman glared accusingly at me, as though the entire predicament of her pregnancy was due to my incompetence.

I then returned to the little license-plate-sized board with a variety of plastic circles representing cervixes in various stages of dilation and practiced sticking my fingers in the holes. Eventually, one day, cervical dilation would become an easy measurement to check; currently it was a major source of discomfiture for me. Again, I know it was an infantile defense, but I thought it unfair to be harshly judged when the women in the group had the advantage of being able to grope their own cervixes and figure out what the hell we were trying to find in the first place.

From those early days of confusion I determined it was always better to be conservative with measurements and not set any expectations. A lot of interns I would work with later in residency would stretch the cervix, thus measuring a falsely increased dilation. The patient would be told their labor was progressing and feel quite happy. Then I would re-check to see if there had actually been any changes and break the bad news. But this was early days in my cervical measuring skills.

As the month progressed, we students were advised to practice exams on women with epidurals who would not be so uncomfortable during our learning phase. Initially I felt this encouragement to check every woman with an epidural as barbaric, but I would attempt a measurement and then the nurse would repeat the exam as the patient looked at me unsure as to why she had to endure this invasive exam twice. I had, after all, been introduced as a doctor (a small fib to boost students' self-esteem), not as an almost-doctor with faulty measuring skills who required a nurse to check his abilities.

There were other ways of determining if a woman was in labor or needed to be admitted to deliver her baby, such as if her water had actually broken. More often than not, the broken water turned out to be due to incontinence and resulted in her going home again. There were other high-risk reasons a woman might be admitted, but cervical dilation and broken water were the most common things we checked for in a straightforward pregnancy.

If the pregnant woman turned out to actually be in labor, she would be checked into a delivery room and we started the paperwork process. Just like the other exciting fields of medicine, obstetrics requires an enormous amount of note writing. I'd record her entire pregnancy history and then use an ultrasound machine to make sure the baby's head was facing down, and not his foot or buttock—you wanted the newborn to dive into life headfirst.

Then we waited.

For hours.

Every two hours I would put the gloves back on and, recheck everything, and record a set of information: cervical dilation, how far the baby's head had descended, the baby's heart rate, the rate and quality of uterus contractions, the patient's pain and temperature. Doctors used the information in these notes to determine when to use medications to augment labor, when to consider a C-section, and when to recognize a trend in the mother's rising temperature and consider whether to start her on antibiotics. Basically it was cover-your-ass time. More importantly, it granted the students and residents another reason not to sleep.

During those hours everybody sat outside the delivery rooms and stared at the monitors displaying the baby's heart rate and the mother's contractions. Like watching stock market tickers and a pot of water not yet boiling, it was mesmerizing, as though staring at the monitor would help produce results. We watched for patterns: are the contractions strong enough and frequent enough to push a baby down the canal, i.e. was labor progressing? We watched the infant's heart rate to make sure it was high enough and not showing signs of distress or fatigue; for example, it was normal for the heart rate to dip down during a contraction, but damn well better come back up afterwards unless the infant wanted a parade of nurses and doctors to march into the exam room and threaten to get out some forceps.

When the woman's cervix was fully dilated it was time for her to start pushing. The first times I announced it was time to start pushing I was under the crazy illusion that a baby would be imminently delivered. I pulled out the delivery cart stocked with all the towels and tools to cut the umbilical cord, put on a cape and gown and gloves, and stood dressed and ready for superhero action (I am kidding about the cape). I watched the monitor excitedly for the next contraction while a much more relaxed nurse looked on impassively.

And then we waited...

And waited...

And waited...

Until, it happened...a contraction!

I rapidly spouted orders to the family members to take up their assigned positions. With military precision, Aunt Marcie and Heather, the mother's cute friend, held up the patient's legs.

I ordered the soon to not-be-pregnant woman to take a big breath, tuck her head to her chest, and push with all her might for, "One, two, three...ten seconds...OK, big breath, and again! One, two...." I was anxious, ready to deliver this baby. I had been up all night with these people; I felt part of the family. They would probably invite me over for christenings, birthdays, and the child's wedding.

Another contraction and I had her repeat the pushes. Finally we saw the top of the baby's head, a two-centimeter patch of fuzzy hair. It was happening, life was happening! A few pushes later and things were really moving along; the fuzzy patch was almost an eighth of a centimeter bigger—maybe.

The resident wandered in to see what was going on.

"She's delivering," I proudly announced, as though I had anything to do with the process.

The resident told the woman "Good work" and just as casually wandered out.

Thirty minutes later I was still in the room, wearing my hot, shower curtain-like gown and gloves, sweating, looking at that tuft of hair and watching the monitor to make sure the heart rate was OK. It was approaching 5:45 a.m. and regretably I had to leave to go check on all the postpartum women who had already delivered their babies. I had the mother push one more time, hopeful of a sudden decision by the child to enter the world into my awaiting hands; but the coy and teasing tuft of hair pushed out and then disappeared back inside again.

I stripped off the gown and sweaty gloves and ran to examine the patients as quickly as I could. An hour later I ran back into the room ready to complete the delivery. And there to my cuckolded surprise sat the happy mother in bed holding her newborn child.

I looked at the smiling resident who had delivered the baby. The family was congratulating him for his fine work: Aunt Marcie giving him gifts, the Grandfather placed a cigar in his scrub pocket, and the cute friend, Heather, appeared to pass him her phone number.

I looked back at the new mother in bed and wanted to say, "You couldn't wait? I thought we had something, me and you." But the fickle woman was preoccupied with her new baby and didn't have time for a jealous medical student.

During those times when I was actually present for the delivery, I watched amazed as the exhausted woman's pushes forced the tuft of hair to slowly grow. At first I was shocked at how large the head became, bigger and bigger until I stood in awe. I had to snap out of the stupor because it was my job to control the head from popping out like a cork under pressure; otherwise, the sudden expulsion of the head could tear a laceration in the vagina.

Regardless of my help, the head would come out and we (there would be an attending or resident doctor present and caring for most of the delivery) would suction out the nose and mouth with a plastic tube (welcome to the world, little one). Next I would stand by, hoping the kid's shoulder would deliver (we had been warned about the dangers of shoulder dystocia, a potentially dangerous situation when the infant's shoulder gets stuck behind the mother's pubic bone and prevents the baby from being delivered—but I'll save shoulder dystocia for stories in residency), followed by the rest of the slippery fellow sliding out and crying, along with the mother and father. I would then clamp and cut the cord, pass off the kid to a nursery team, and find I was crying with everybody else. No, not really, but I heard it happened.

Then we waited to deliver the placenta. This was usually a moment of downtime where the exhausted woman lay back while her baby was dried and washed. The doctor and I stood between her legs, waiting to deliver the placenta, and discussing the delivery, like a post-mission debriefing. Then the red blob came out and we checked to make sure it was all there. And that was the simplest of deliveries. I will go into more details on complicated deliveries during the residency years, although one deserves an honorable mention here: The world's fastest caesarian section.

The OB I was working with one day happened to be a close family friend of the woman delivering. Throughout the labor he kept very cool, stopping in to chat with the family and checking on the patient's progression—which was non-existent. He jokingly told me to start doing a better job and reassured the family that everything was fine. And it was, for a few hours. Then the baby got fed up with the pushing and decided to drop his heart rate, just to show us how much he wanted to stay in his own personal hot tub.

The doctor responded to this hostile act by calmly deciding it was time to yank the kid out with forceps. And being a smart OB attending, who was friends with the family, he decided to do so in the OR.

As we wheeled the pregnant woman out of the room, her grandmother grabbed me by the arm. "Take care of my little girl, please," she implored me. Not that I really had anything to do with the event besides wheeling her granddaughter down the hallway, but suddenly I felt like I was supposed to take over if things started to go poorly.

Fortunately, in the OR everybody was very calm and I found no reason to knock the attending out of the way to put my yet-undiscovered obstetric skills into action for the grandmother's sake. The attending assured the mother yet again that he was just being overly cautious by being in the OR rather than the delivery room. He placed the forceps on the baby's head and gently exerted some mild traction.

The baby's heart rate nosedived.

The doctor shouted, "Let's go!"

A samurai katana blade flashed through the air and the pregnant belly was sliced open.

In seven seconds flat the baby was out and passed to the nursery team. The attending, now wearing a kimono, raised his hands overhead as though to celebrate a calf roping record.

Fastest delivery in the West, and of course, I'm joking about the kimono.

P.S. the mother already had an epidural placed, so she did not feel a thing.

But that excitement was rare. For the next weeks either I spent the night in the hospital or I got up at 4:30 a.m. and drove into a dark parking lot, walked up one flight of stairs, and checked off which patients I needed to visit before the terror of morning rounds.

The morning rounds process in OB had its own language and its own set of key questions. You started by determining how the woman had delivered her baby. A straightforward delivery was called a normal-spontaneous-vaginal-delivery, or NSVD. But was it spontaneous if we had given her medications to induce or augment delivery? There were forceps deliveries, vacuum deliveries, deliveries with and without lacerations and the complications of the deliveries themselves. If the patient had experienced heavy vaginal bleeding after delivery and received a blood transfusion, and you did not supply this key fact in rounds, you were executed.

Or, even worse, in front of the host of nurses, nursing students, medical students, and residents you would be publicly humiliated with the words, "Your work is not acceptable."

After deciphering how the woman had delivered, you next had to figure out which pregnancy this was for her—including abortions, pre-term deliveries, and miscarriages. Not as simple a task as it sounds, especially when working with non-English speaking patients at five in the morning.

Have you ever tried miming, "Did you have any pre-term deliveries or miscarriages?" to a Romanian-speaking woman?

I have. Neither of us gained anything from that conversation.

Then there were the key questions for the postpartum mother: "Is your pain controlled?"

The majority of Spanish speaking women would reply that they were fine and could they please go home now.

The majority of non-Hispanic or non-Polynesian women under age twenty-two would ask for stronger narcotics and more frequently, please. Then it was a quick rundown of key questions: "Did you urinate? How heavy is your vaginal bleeding? Are you dizzy? Any shortness of breath? Any leg pain? And what form of birth control would you like to use for the next months?"

Miming out that last question to non-English speakers always provided moments of embarrassment, confusion and hilarity for everybody in the room at 6 a.m.

If the patient had undergone a Caesarian-section, then you also asked if she was passing gas or having a bowel movement yet? Just casual, run of the mill, everyday questions.

A quick listen to the lungs, an uncomfortable push on her stomach to make sure the uterus felt firm, and squeeze the calf muscles to make sure there were no blood clots developing.

If a mother with a C-section was going home, you got to remove the staples holding her belly together and glue on some steri-strips. They never said thank you for that fun bit of morning arts and crafts.

That's what happens on the postpartum floor of the hospital early every morning.

After seeing all the patients, we convened at the "Big Board" to discuss any patients remaining in labor from the previous night. Most women did deliver at nighttime or into the early morning—and full moons did cause mayhem, not superstition, they really did create labor chaos.

Then the moment of truth as the medical students, residents, interns, and attending physicians gathered around a table and the students were ordered to recite their postpartum patient notes. To add to the pressure of being front and center on stage we were also expected to deliver all the information in one big breath of air, saying everything as fast as possible.

Inhale deeply and: "Miss. Escocharria is a sixteen-year-old G2P1001 postpartum day number two status-post NSVD at thirty-seven weeks whose pain is well controlled is tolerating liquids and solids urinating without difficulty ambulating no respiratory symptoms and would like to go home today she was afebrile vital signs stable lungs clear regular rate and rhythm abdomen had firm fundus two centimeters below the umbilicus she is O+ plans to breast feed use the mini pill plan to discharge today or tomorrow."

And then I waited to be grilled about the one vital piece of information that I had missed and they had somehow deciphered via my eloquent James Joyce monologue.

If we survived rounding and filling out endless stacks of paper work to discharge the patients, then we returned to the labor and delivery deck to help care for more mothers in the endless cycle of labor and delivery.

I endured those weeks with very little sleep, worked hard, and despite not impressing Dr. Sutherland with my brazen habit of snoring in front of him during teaching sessions, made an otherwise good impression as a decent medical student—all of which culminated on my final call night.

During my last night a woman's labor was not going well at all—she was in pain and the baby was not coming down the canal for delivery.

Derek, the chief resident again that night, pulled me aside and said, "John, I want you to take care of this patient, not the family practice (FP) resident. I trust you more than her. Can you do that? Deliver her start to finish?"

Of course I could. So I bumped the FP resident (awkward) and took over the whole situation. I sat with the pregnant mother for hours; at one point convincing Derek that the patient was making progress and did not need a C-section. I sat with her, encouraging her to push with every contraction until it was time for me to round in the morning. I rushed through rounds and then ran back to her room, figuring I had missed the grand finale as usual.

But I must be improving as a student because for once, I arrived back just in time to put on gown and gloves and join Derek between the patient's legs. And then Derek stepped aside to let me run the delivery.

The mother pushed and I controlled the infant's head as it began to enter the world. Baby's shoulders were delivered easily, and the baby slipped into my arms. Umbilical cord clamped and cut; baby's nose suctioned; baby dried and wrapped in blankets; baby passed to waiting nursery team.

That was my graduation delivery: No real drama or excitement, just a calm delivery, which is what it was supposed to be. And I felt confident in what I was doing the entire time— which of course signaled it was time to move to a new service, in this case, gynecology, where I would once again be at a loss for what to say or do.

GYNECOLOGY

THE ART OF WATERSKIING

After delivering babies with the obstetrics team, we were transferred to the flip side of the female pelvic service, the gynecology (GYN) team. For this surgical rotation, my student team moved to a different hospital with all sorts of perks: flattering green scrubs; not having to be in the hospital until 6:30 a.m.; and best of all, free bagels every morning and free sandwiches at lunchtime to keep us animals fed. The small things made the biggest differences.

When I started the rotation, gynecology team members kept asking if I liked to waterski. I had only tried it a couple of times, was miserable at it, but thought it was nice of them to keep asking. Apparently a lot of water-skiers go into gynecology.

I dropped the social banter briefly to learn about our new routine. Not much instruction was given; we were told to simply sign up for posted surgeries and then go stand in the respective OR for several hours. That was the extent of our training and instruction: sign in and show up.

The majority of the gynecological cases were either

removing uteruses (hysterectomies) or exploring a uterus to locate the source of pelvic pain—usually blamed on endometriosis, a growth of uterine tissue outside the uterus that was treated by cauterization.

Most of the patients with pelvic pain were back to try the same procedure for a second, third, or even fourth time after the previous attempts had failed to produce any relief. One either had to question the sanity of patients opting for "third times a charm" surgery, or applaud both their optimism, and the doctor's enthusiasm, in getting them to try one more time. And lastly, gynecological surgery was often life-saving in that it enabled the diagnosis and treatment of invasive cancerous tumors.

We medical students introduced ourselves to the crew of residents, nurses, and attending physicians, all of whom considered us, at best, to be in the way. Two gynecology surgeons, in particular, had gained the reputation of being such terrors with medical students that we were banned from ever working with them.

On only one other occasion did I know of students and residents being instructed not to work with an attending physician. That particular case involved the general surgeon who was actually in charge of teaching the surgical residents. He had lost his cool in the OR and started kicking things, including the phone off the wall. The chief surgical resident made an executive decision that he would not allow his interns to work under such abusive conditions. A bold statement for a resident to make and it made a lasting impression on me that residents were human too and had some basic rights, like protection from abuse.

On my first day joining the gynecology service, I signed up for a posted hysterectomy surgery, scrubbed in, and walked into my assigned operating room for the day. Standing at the table were the two infamous doctors I was not supposed to be working with for my own safety.

But there was no turning back as the larger of the two saw me balking in the doorway and shouted, "What's your name?"

"John, the medical student."

"Well, don't get in the way."

"I rarely do."

He pointed to the unconscious woman lying with her legs spread on the operating table and ordered, "Stick your fingers in there and tell me what you think."

I proceeded to do a pelvic exam on the unconscious woman.

Apparently my technique was too gentle as the attending urged me on, saying, "Come on, get in there, she's not going to feel anything. Whatta'ya feel?"

"Uh…a mass?"

I had never felt a vaginal mass, but it was the only thing I could think of since we were supposed to be removing masses in gynecology.

"Jesus Christ," he muttered disappointedly. "Forty-year old-virgin. What a waste, let's get going."

Looking at the patient, lying there, unconscious, I was uncertain if the attending was disappointed in the patient's celibacy or my lack of anything resembling gynecological knowledge.

Either way, learning or not, the attitude felt a bit repugnant. But at the time, as an intimidated student, I went through the service with the primary goal of surviving, i.e. avoid getting noticed or kicked out. Perhaps other students were confidently stepping into surgeries, asking questions, rebuking physicians for their crudeness…I was not that student. I was still lost in my underdog stature as the head-injured, liberal arts student waiting to be recognized as an imposter and escorted out of the hospital.

I won't deny there were often crude jokes from certain surgeons or anesthesia doctors…but these were rare and never intended maliciously; it was humor, occasionally dark humor, which got everyone through long hours; bad outcomes; uncertainty; and lack of sleep. Underneath it all, I believe, were genuinely caring people who were forced to put up a screen to deal with the sheer quantity of patients and the inability to cure everyone. They strove to prevent emotional reality from destroying them mentally as they faced patient death, frustration, and stress-spiking surgeries all day, every day. We've all experienced humor getting us through tough times. That said, I doubt this attitude is tolerated any longer in the post #MeToo era.

Commentary over, we now return to our regularly scheduled gynecological procedure, which is most likely, drumroll please, a hysterectomy. Hysterectomies were by far the most common item on the surgery schedule, the only variant being: *Vaginal or Abdominal? You want ovaries with that?* Gynecology seemed to be principally focused about the removal of uteruses. It was as if these physicians, who had been trained to get babies out of the uterus as Obstetricians, then had to make sure it never happened again. The other common GYN surgery, as mentioned, was searching for the source of a woman's pelvic pain with an exploratory laparoscopy, literally exploring a woman's uterus.

"Exploratory" procedures always sounded like we were voyaging off on an expedition to map the Yukon and spot Bigfoot. Just as in those adventures, the object of our search proved elusive and we rarely found what we had set out to discover in the first place.

I had three roles to master when scrubbed into gynecological surgeries. The first was speaking. I was to answer any questions thrown in my direction: anatomical questions from the resident, musical questions from the anesthesiologist, and a variety of queries from the attending physicians.

The attending's questions ranged from: "Where the hell did you come from?" to "What the hell are you going to do with your life?" to "Why the hell are you in medicine?", and all the way to "Hell, can't you hold that retractor like a man?"

My second role during surgery, was not answering questions, but counting—counting all the way to ten.

Twenty years of education and I was charged with proving I could still count to ten. Counting to ten was critical, as the surgeons cauterized the potential source of a women's pelvic pain for that exact ten count, historically delegated to medical students. I'm not sure what they did if students were absent; cancel the surgery, I imagine.

Medical school had not trained me for exploratory laparoscopies, and, as mentioned, the introduction to the gynecology service had been non-existent, so you might imagine the immense pressure I felt when I was told to count to ten. I'm not joking; I actually thought they were mocking me that first time, attempting to trip me up with some obscure gynecology request. But I successfully counted to ten, albeit tentatively, and realized that I'd finally found something I was competent at in medicine, counting.

My gynecological mastery culminated on a day when, to really spice things up, I was asked to count to ten in Spanish. I rose to the challenge, *sin problemo*.

Then they tried challenging me to count in French—*Et ce n'etait pas un problème*. I had lived in France after college surviving on stolen green beans.

"How about German?" dared a nurse. I had once asked a high school teacher to teach me German, so I knew that one, too, along with how to ask for some beers (*Zwei bier bitte?*), how to say the window is closed (das fenster ist geschlossen.), and how to sing Beethoven's *Ode to Joy*.

Then the scrub-tech double-dared me, "What about Japanese?"

Non-plussed, I counted off, "ichi, ni, san…" all the way to ten in Japanese. (A Japanese teammate on my high school soccer team had fortuitously taught me to count to ten.)

Finally the anesthesiologist threw down the latex gauntlet: "Do it in Polish."

Six months before I started medical school I had lived in Poland, overseeing a financial blunder that involved me learning how to count to ten and beyond.

Without missing a beat I counted, "jeden, dwa, trzy…" all the way to ten in Polish.

Game, set, and match.

Suddenly I was the new hero at Court and the attending and anesthesiologist started talking to me as though I was a regular human being, not some ragamuffin crawling out of a pile of crap; it was truly my *Slumdog Millionaire* moment.

For almost a minute, I actually began to relax, but then the pesky resident jealously chimed in, "So, tell us the advantages of a vaginal hysterectomy over an abdominal approach?"

I wanted to pipe up, *"Hey geeky resident, weren't you paying attention? I can count to ten in different languages."* But I was feeling lucky. I decided the resident was trying to trick me, and threw out, "There are none?"

Not even close.

The resident shook his head: "You might want to study a bit more before scrubbing in. why don't you tell us tomorrow."

My newly made counting friends all looked away unwilling to defend my ignorance.

You may wonder what else I did on this rotation besides playing Ask Jeeves, counting to ten, and confirming the resident's suspicions that I didn't study enough. Well, my third role, the truly important part of my medical training, was holding retractors.

Retractors are metal surgical tools used to pull skin or tissue out of the way for surgeons to operate with a clear field of view. Medical students are trained to hold retractors and stay out of the way themselves. For what seemed like hours I held onto metal handles that were attached to large metal retractors that stretched open the patient's belly. I just held on, leaned way back with my arms extended, and got out of the way so the surgeons could work.

This enviable task solved the mysterious abundance of water-skiers in gynecology. Yes, herein lay the fun sport of "waterskiing," leaning back and holding those retractors until your shoulders were falling off.

Every once in a while somebody would ask if I knew what artery they were trying to avoid cutting. I couldn't see past the backs of surgeon's heads and just threw out guesses. Since we assisted on the same surgeries over and over, after several weeks I learned the correct answers because they asked the same questions every time. And as usual, the day I finally guessed three correct answers in a row was my last day on the gynecology service—which was great because the waterskiing was killing my shoulders.

GENERAL SURGERY

RECTAL ROCKETS AND WHY WE EAT OUR VEGETABLES

There's a rivalry between residents: Surgery vs. Medicine. It's not quite on par with Yankees vs. Red Sox, or Tottenham vs. Arsenal for you English football fans—in fact, it's not really much of a rivalry at all—except to surgical residents. Surgery, as the name states, refers to anyone performing surgery, while "medicine" refers to the rest of the bozos pretending that they're doctors in the eyes of surgical residents. Surgeons genuinely expected themselves to work harder and longer than anyone else, and to be the most intelligent doctors in the hospital.

This assertion was critical to understand as a medical student because it informed your answer to a surgical resident asking, "What are you going into?" This seemingly innocuous question, regarding what residency path you were considering, had one correct answer unless you wanted to be ignored and likely mocked for the entire rotation as being a "medicine" wimp.

The general surgery rotation was rumored to chew up medical students and spit them out sleepless, tearful, fearful wretches begging for mercy. If it didn't, you might have the makings of a surgeon. My girlfriend (yes, the same top-of-her-class student) had loved the challenge of surgical rotations. More than any other rotation, surgery demanded you be on your toes all the time, studying large volumes of surgery texts in non-existent spare time, studying specific surgery cases right before you scrubbed in; planning to never sleep; and saying good-bye to your friends, to eating, and to anything humane. You lived and breathed surgery for eight weeks. My pathologically hardworking girlfriend had been totally in her element.

Meanwhile, surgery residents scoff at any such melodrama. They love what they do and compete to see who can work longer, sleep less, and save more lives. These residents had a simple survival mantra: "See a bed, sleep in it; See a toilet, pee in it; See a donut, eat a donut."

We students were just starting to realize you could survive any crazy schedule for several weeks. And like the frog in a pot of slowly heating water, did not feel our simmering relationship with sanity or civilization boiling away. As you went further into training, your mind warped and you believed that those months without regular sleep, without seeing sunlight or friends, was normal.

When you had an entire weekend off, you were incredulous that some people had *every* weekend off. *What the hell did they do with all that free time??*

If you answered, "Study surgery," then congratulations, you're delirious and considered worthy of a surgical residency.

At that time I was happy to work hard with long hours that prevented my mind dwelling on the loss of my friend a few months prior. I had signed up for the "blue team," wanting to be challenged. The blue team was a notoriously hardworking crew with the chairman of surgery as one of the attending physicians. If you wanted to impress the head honcho of surgery and had thoughts of applying to the general surgery residency program, you got yourself on the blue team and worked your ass off. I looked forward to working with him as he had a similar appearance to David Letterman and supposedly tried to stay lighthearted and joking, like his visual counterpart.

But my general surgery future was fortuitously thwarted when a student in my medical class, also wanting to be a surgeon, used subterfuge to change my request so that somehow he was placed on the blue team instead of me.

"But *I* want to be on the blue team," I whined. So we played rock-paper-scissors.

Before we threw out our hands, in one of those time-slowing moments, I remember looking at him and thinking this Machiavellian student will throw paper...and he did.

At the same instant, with time crawling, I thought of my girlfriend, who a year ago had been lauded on the blue team as their top student. She wanted me to experience the blue team and to do well on it, if only for the excellent learning; she was that kind of wonderful student and encouraging friend. I wondered in that instant if she would be disappointed in me as I thrust forward a closed fist.

Yes, I lost to that backstabbing, surgical-wannabe, grinning student. But *just maybe* it was a Freudian throw of "rock" because instead of becoming a whipping boy for the busy blue team at the University Hospital, I was assigned to the green team at the V.A. hospital and concerns of brutally long hours evaporated.

Surgical residents called the V.A. hospital the "VA-Spa." The V.A. schedule, with a smaller patient census, was very relaxed compared to working in other hospitals. We still had long days and call nights in the hospital, but I had gone from weeks of miserable hours to a relatively laidback month with happy surgical residents and cheery attending physicians.

Please understand that everything is relative, so by *laidback* I mean, we once actually left the hospital for lunch; and one time we played basketball in the VA gymnasium for almost twelve minutes, once. But those two moments, however brief, were a blissful respite, where for several minutes you could almost stop thinking about surgery.

Otherwise, we were still awake on call nights, working with the same medical residents and attending physicians that worked in the other hospitals, and learning to give the same excellent care that surgeons anywhere expect. We were just allowed to smile once in awhile.

We spent our first two days being oriented, learning what the team expected of us and how to not screw up… sound familiar? We practiced scrubbing into surgeries, a procedure most students messed up repeatedly, which required being yelled at by scrub techs. I'm pretty sure that the ability to humiliate medical students is a requirement on scrub techs' resumes.

Fortunately, I had prior practice being humiliated by scrub techs from my time on the gynecology service where I had repeatedly scrubbed into surgeries every day to remove women's uteruses. I passed the scrub-into-surgery lesson quickly and felt ready to remove gnarled veterans' colons and gallbladders. But first, in order to survive and be productive, we learned what all the operating instruments were called, what to do and not do in the OR, how to find your way through the labyrinth of V.A. tunnels (that had been built to withstand a nuclear freeze), and how to get to the basketball court and cafeteria via those tunnels.

Then it was the first morning of work and we started with rounds—this time rounding on patients that were scheduled for surgery or that had undergone surgery already.

The student's task was to examine assigned patients before the sun came up because then it was time to operate. Surgeons demand efficiency; they want every minute detail of possible importance delivered perfectly, with patient presentations organized and delivered the same way they would expect to hear from anyone weaned on surgery. It was all very formal. The team stood at attention during patient presentations with only the chief resident leaning against the wall (On the OB rotation we had sat slumped over a desk; on medicine we stood shuffling and unkempt). Stethoscopes were put away, not wrapped around our neck as with OB or even worse, medicine people. And we always attended breakfast, lunch, and dinner together.

As for the V.A. food... well, as one resident gleefully pointed out, "It's free." And it was. It was good old American diner food: grits, French toast, and scrambled eggs. And to keep things in perspective, the blue team probably hadn't eaten in days.

My first patient to round on that morning was Mr. Hidashi (he was Hispanic, but had a Japanese-sounding name), who had a problem called entero-fistulas. These were essentially large holes from his body cavity into the outside world. Part of my daily routine was to take all the gauze dressings out from these enormous wounds and replace them with new ones.

Mr. Hidashi had been in the hospital for weeks and was used to the routine. I, however, was not. Not used to finding patients' rooms in a new hospital. Not used to finding hidden stores of dressings and gloves and certainly not used to stuffing gauze into this man's foul-smelling chest wall. He would talk casually about hospital food while I thought to myself: *I bet none of my friends are stuffing gauze into some guy's necrotic chest wall at 6 a.m. every morning.*

Later that afternoon I had a student meeting, and then returned to the hospital at 5 p.m. to stay overnight as I was on-call. I found my team preparing to start a surgery. After the previous month long redundancy of removing uteruses, I was excited to finally be scrubbing in for some new surgery. *This is great*, I thought.

I went through the diligent scrubbing technique: surgical booties and hat on, wash hands, open the surgical scrub brush, use the sponge to wash everything from fingers to forearm, then scrub each side of each finger ten times with the brush, especially under the nails. Rinse hands, then rinse forearms, holding them upright so water from my arm did not run down and contaminate my sterile hands. I walked into the OR, properly holding my dripping hands upright, and a scrub nurse held out a welcoming sterile green towel to dry my hands before wrapping me in a gown and placing sterile gloves on my hands. I was being treated like part of the team, a real doctor, even.

I turned towards the center of the room where my chief resident was prepping the patient for surgery. Lying there, sedated on the operating table, was a woman. I knew she was a woman because I had been operating on the gynecology service for the last month and was quite adept at recognizing gender specifics.

Of all the surgeries, in all the operating rooms, this patient comes to the V.A. for a hysterectomy.

Well shit guys; go home, I can do this one blindfolded.

In a nonchalant, almost bored manner, I nailed every single question asked by the attending, resident, and anesthesiologist. Once everybody mistakenly assumed I was a surgical genius, we chatted about more casual interests and the team seemed doubly impressed to find out I had interests outside of medicine. Suddenly we were talking like old friends at a bar, saddled up to the operating table, wielding surgical tools without pretensions. This was another great lesson—if you started with a good reputation, you could usually hold on to it unless you really screwed up. But if you started off on the wrong foot, it was really hard to shake it off. There was no award for most improved medical student.

The hysterectomy was routine and we scrubbed out in time to grab dinner at the cafeteria. The chief resident turned out to be a very relaxed, friendly, and athletic guy—a trail runner, skier, and rock-climber who also enjoyed long hours in the hospital. He and his surgical buddies would routinely stay awake for 36 hours in the hospital, leave work, and instead of catching up on sleep, go for a 20-mile run until 3 a.m., then sleep, and be back at work at 6 a.m. looking refreshed. If they had more hours off duty, they ran ultra-marathons while discussing surgery.

Later, that first night on-call, the chief resident called me back into the operating room. The woman we had operated on several hours ago, the routine hysterectomy patient, had dropped her blood pressure and was bleeding vaginally. The two of us took her back to the OR, cut her open again, and were surprised to discover a lot of blood pooling in her abdomen.

In a somewhat amused and relaxed voice, the resident evaluated the mess and surmised, "Huh. Well... it was dry when we closed." He found the site of bleeding, tied off the naughty leaking blood vessel and allowed me to close her up again.

("Closing up" refers to suturing and stapling closed the abdomen after it has been cut open for surgery).

After a month of being third-assist on many, many hysterectomy cases, this was the first complication I had ever seen.

One benefit of the V.A. was that the residents were allowed to perform surgeries while the attending physicians billed for the work without being present. This little ripple in the system has since been changed so that the attending must be in the general vicinity of the OR, i.e. *preferably* in the building, not just within a proximity of less than seven golf courses.

At times we actually had an attending scrub in, usually working between several operating rooms. Sometimes they just showed up for a quick guest appearance before lunch. The fun of having no attending present was kind of like what happens in any class when the teacher steps out. In this case it meant the residents, if they thought you capable, allowed the students to do some simple surgery rather than forcing us to hold retractors for hours. Not that holding retractors didn't have its merits; my grip strength was really improving, but it was difficult to stay awake when you were under-slept, and standing for hours with nothing to do but lean back on those retractor handles.

The following night our intern, happy to be on a relaxing rotation relative to the rest of his hellacious intern year, was kicking back on call when the code alarm went off. He ran to the coding patient's room where he found an unconscious patient who had undergone carotid artery surgery earlier that day. The surgery site had started bleeding internally and the resultant swelling was cutting off the blood supply to his brain. The intern cut open the surgery site and tried to relieve the pressure—but it was too late and the patient died.

Complications were adding up at the Va-Spa.

A few nights later I was on call again and the night's slumber was ruined because a patient in the surgical ICU (SICU) was getting sicker. His leg had become infected and was not responding to antibiotic therapy. Amputating his leg seemed the only way to save his body from overwhelming sepsis.

The patient's family had previously opposed any amputation, as the patient was a young guy. But it was the weekend and we were unable to contact his family. Our team found the patient unconscious from the worsening infection. As usual, the attending physicians were nowhere to be found on the weekend, so the chief residents pondered the options and agreed that the only way to keep the patient alive would be to remove the infection, i.e. cut off the leg. So they did.

A tourniquet was applied, the meat and bone sawed through, and I was handed the amputated leg and told to take it downstairs. Wandering the nuclear freeze-resistant halls with a hefty garbage bag I pondered, *I bet none of my friends are wandering around hospital tunnels at 2 a.m. on a Saturday night carrying an amputated leg.*

Now for a reassuring aside: For those of you now concerned about ever showing up at a V.A. hospital, rest well knowing that, while did I lump these complications together, the number of complications at the V.A. was far fewer than what was seen at the larger, busier hospitals, just a matter of patient volume. The care at the V.A. remains excellent.

Besides hospital surgery, the V.A. rotation included the "Lump and Bump" clinic. Two afternoons a week, instead of cutting and stapling intestines back together (oh yes, read on), we examined patients and determined who needed surgery or who needed to have a lump removed right there in clinic. The one patient I remember quite well was an older fellow, Alfred, a farmer from Wyoming, with a small bump on his forehead.

I consulted my chief resident, who agreed I should cut Alfred's forehead open and take out the bump. So, I did. An ugly-looking round blob popped out and I sewed the forehead back together again.

The following week the pathology report came back and the blob turned out to be some cancer-oma—which meant it was a good thing we had taken it out.

Unfortunately, the margins of the tumor were not clear, i.e. I had not removed all the cancer. So when Alfred returned from the farm to have his sutures removed, I told him we had removed a cancerous tumor, which was good, but now needed to cut the rest out. This time I cut a bigger incision in his forehead, removed lots of the surrounding tissue, sewed him up again and sent him home.

The following week the pathology report returned stating that I had not yet removed the entire tumor—there were still margins of tissue with cancer. So I called Alfred back to the hospital, yet again. How embarrassing.

At the same time I was not sure how much more tissue I could cut away; there was only so much I could remove from Alfred's head without a decapitation, which seemed to cross the boundaries of the Hippocratic oath.

At this juncture I was also unsure how much confidence the patient had in my abilities, so I asked my chief resident to accompany me. Once again I cleaned Alfred's forehead and injected a local anesthetic before cutting a huge incision deep into his forehead and removing more soft tissue. The chief resident just kept shrugging his shoulders as if to say, *cut out more, why not?* So we took out as much surrounding tissue as seemed feasible.

Removing tissue had its drawbacks. Tissue is filled with blood vessels. The more I cut, the more blood spurted and ran everywhere. Smoke now filled the cramped room as I cauterized anything that looked like a bleeding vessel.

And all that time, Alfred was awake, blood running down his face, listening to his wife's reactions to our *Little Shop of Horror* scalping efforts. She backed further and further away from her blood-spattered husband, asking worriedly, "Oh, Alfred, are you OK? Alfred? Are you alright under there?"

My chief resident seemed relaxed, while personally, I started to question if Alfred was going to survive my hackneyed efforts.

But that time we got it all and Alfred walked out several pounds lighter on his toes.

We did have fun on that team: removing gall bladders, removing huge spleens, playing basketball, and repairing many hernias. Before entering the OR, I would quickly review a description of the upcoming procedure in a large textbook of surgeries. A quick refresher was helpful to learn which arteries we would be cutting near, what tissue we would cut through, the statistical prognoses of the disease we were treating, etc., as these were the types of questions we faced during the surgery.

As the team started cutting open a patient, the resident would ask, "What am I cutting through now?" And you would hopefully know the tissue plane.

Then another resident would ask, "Can you name the three other methods for repairing hiatal hernias and why this method is the most common?"

And my answer would be, "No." But the next day, I was expected to have a report with several articles supporting the reason for the Nissan fundoplication wrap being the most common method of repairing a hiatal hernia.

And so it went: study for a surgery, assist on that surgery, and answer related questions, hoping to avoid curveballs, such as Mr. Smithfield eating breakfast.

You would occasionally show up prepared for a specific surgery and discover they had changed the patient operating schedule because Mr. Smithfield, against orders, had decided to eat three helpings of French toast the morning of his scheduled surgery. I couldn't fault Mr. Smithfield; the V.A. French toast was really tasty. Although after several episodes of similar antics from Smithfield, one had to wonder if patients were purposefully sabotaging their surgeries in order to spend more time in the V.A. with free food. So instead of repairing Smithfield's hernia we would be doing a colectomy with colostomy on Mr. Withers (taking out his cancerous colon and attaching a colostomy bag on his stomach).

The problem was that I was ready to answer hernia questions that had nothing to do with questions regarding Mr. Withers and his colon cancer.

As we started cutting Withers, a resident would start the interrogation routine: "Ok medical student, why don't you tell us the major risk factors for colon cancer and the treatment options?"

I would reply, "Good question. How about I tell you the borders of an indirect hernia?" And the resident would frown at my ignorance; completely unaware that Smithfield's gluttony was the cause of my apparent ineptitude.

Fortunately the surgical residents' moods were easily lifted when the time came to cut out the colon and they were handed some newfangled Ginzu-colon-stapler-cutter-tool-in-one. There was gleeful skipping and dancing in the operating room whenever new toys were unwrapped for surgeries. One friend was actually a drug company representative for a device called the "rectal rocket."

After repairing hernias, resecting colon cancer was probably the most common surgery we performed that month.

Colon cancer surgery results in patients having colostomy bags. I could write more about colostomy bags, but bags of shit are really not that interesting. Their best use is probably being displayed to schoolchildren to scare them into eating their vegetables.

Colon cancer is quite prevalent, so there was a lot of time, money and research that went into tools for cutting out the colon and rectum and closing it off. Trickier than it sounds, and it usually required, after the colon was cut away, that a junior resident crawl under the operating field to make sure the rectal area was properly closed off, and then they poked through the abdomen to make a colostomy site.

I realize the discussion of colons, rectums, and feces is not really all that pleasant—but such is the focus of medicine and especially surgery.

Speaking of rectums, one afternoon, post-call night, we were paged to the ER to evaluate a patient with a rectal abscess. The entire team had completed their work so we all headed down to see the patient together.

We arrived in the ER exam room and discovered the patient had taken off for a stroll, so we waited. Several minutes later, limping towards us, we see a 5'4" squirrelly-looking guy, wearing an orthopedic boot on one leg and an oversized baseball cap tilted to one side of his head; there was also a wooden stick poking out of his neck that kept knocking the hat off his head as he limped towards us. To top off his crazy appearance, he had very lively strabismus. Strabismus, also known as lazy eye, meant his eyes didn't quite function together. In this case his eyes seemed to be continually spinning in different directions. Our patient was the type of guy that if you saw walking towards you down a sidewalk, would make you cross to the other side of the road without making eye contact.

In the exam room I was less intrigued about his rectal abscess and more concerned with what looked like an arrow sticking out of his neck.

The resident was equally puzzled and finally asked, "Do you know you have a stick in your neck?" Because he did appear to be the type of oddball that might walk around for years without realizing there was something impaling his skin until he turned up on the evening news. Turned out it was just a long stick he kept in the back of his shirt in case he was itchy.

Our fears allayed, we were then treated to a three-minute oration on his need to have a back-scratching stick ready at all times. A painful oration to listen to, but it relieved our fears of taking him to the OR to remove an ill-shot arrow. After getting through all such pleasantries, we told him we needed to look at his rectal abscess.

At this point he informed us that, "Last time someone touched my ass was 'Nam and I killed 'em. I'll kill any of you touches my ass."

The addition of a death threat did nothing to increase our already booming desire to examine his rectum (that's sarcasm, just to be clear). It did, however, open the floodgates of the post-call night, sleep-deprived giggles we had all been politely repressing since he walked towards us.

Our chief resident calmly explained that we had no sexual desires towards him and that we just needed to see the area that was hurting.

After twenty minutes of hearing our continual promises that we had no hanky-panky planned while examining him, he graciously dropped his pants, allowing us to admire the red painful abscess between his buttocks.

Our resident explained that we needed to numb the area with a needle and drain the infected wound. The patient quickly retorted that he had kicked the shit out of the last doctor that touched him with a needle.

The entire team was already having a difficult time taking anything he said seriously due to his spinning eyes and remarkable resemblance to a miniature Robin Williams without teeth.

Again it took time to convince him that he needed the infection drained and he finally agreed, insisting, however, that he needed no numbing medication because he had been in the military and was trained to handle any pain, including torture.

Fine.

We agreed to use minimal anesthetic. I helped set up all the necessary instruments for draining the abscess while the patient rambled on about his pain tolerance, how tough he was, and how many people he had "kicked the shit out of."

The chief resident was careful to warn the patient of what he was doing, "I'm going to clean the area with some surgical scrub, ready?"

"Go ahead, I can handle pain."

"It's just a sponge with water and soap."

"OK, but no funny business."

The skin was "prepped" clean for the procedure.

Then our chief prepared to inject lidocaine to numb the skin.

"I'm going to inject some numbing medicine with a needle."

"Go ahead, I told you, I can handle torture."

The resident poked the wound with a needle and the patient immediately screamed so loudly that we all bolted from the room terrified he was about to start swinging.

The patient refused any further treatment.

While our team enjoyed the time together, it was still long hours of examining patients, paperwork, and studying, when time permitted. The residents however, had the added pressure of keeping patients alive.

Through the daily fears of what the cafeteria would attempt to pass off as food, the challenge of finding gauze to stuff into Mr. Hidashi's chest, finding a minute to study before entering the OR, and finding clean scrubs, it was easy to forget that there were people actually concerned with living through our learning process.

So in order to keep residents from forgetting about the importance of not screwing up, there was a weekly conference that all surgery residents had to survive. It was a brutal interrogation called the "Morbidity and Mortality conference" (M&M). Throughout the week the residents in all the teaching hospitals recorded anything that went wrong with patients, such as dying or bleeding complications requiring a return to the OR.

Then all the residents and all the students assembled in a conference room with the entire host of attending physicians, and meticulously reviewed each case. These conferences were great for students because you were not expected to say anything; instead, we got to eat snacks and watch the fireworks.

A resident from each surgical service stood and presented cases—what happened and what went wrong. Attending physicians would then fire off questions regarding why a case had been handled a certain way and the residents were forced to defend their actions. This was serious accountability for why patients had become sick, had an amputation, or died.

The attending physicians would basically force residents to accept how they had killed the patient—all for the sake of teaching them in an unforgettable manner that would prevent that mistake from ever happening again.

Humor was not completely alien to this usually hostile accountability reckoning, such as when my chief resident needed to discuss why we had returned to the operating room for the lady with the hysterectomy who started bleeding. The bleeding complication could have been more dangerous and returning to the OR meant putting the patient at risk with all the possible complications of surgery.

"Well... it was dry when we closed," he sheepishly grinned, admitting our blunder. But he was a well-liked, senior resident who could get away with droll humor and fortunately the case had ended well.

The most entertaining cases, however, involved attending physicians being forced to defend their actions with each other. While the residents were held accountable for the complications, the attending surgeons were ultimately responsible for everything that happened to the patients. So when one attending attacked a resident's shoddy care of a patient, it was an indirect attack on his fellow attending. We heard of fabled M&M conferences with surgeons leaping over seats, launching themselves at each other's jugular, being held back from going fist-a-cuffs.

And from what I understood we were experiencing a very tame M&M environment compared to what are known as "malignant" teaching hospitals where shouting and crying was commonplace and residents left conferences in need of compassionate therapy.

Fortunately the V.A. hospital's attendings were the most relaxed of all the general surgery attendings. They never grilled us too harshly, and actually seemed to enjoy working with us.

One big reason for their relaxed attitude was that they only showed up for part of the day. The new rule I mentioned has since been clarified to state that the attending physician actually be present for all surgeries. At that time the rules had been roughly translated as: "The attending should be present in the operating room at some point during the week." The chief residents, mere months from graduating, were practically attending surgeons themselves.

There was one exception to my otherwise blissful existence on surgery and that was my temporary transfer for several days onto the "gold" team. The gold team was the vascular surgery team and they operated more like surgery teams at the university hospital; i.e. they worked harder than I had become accustomed to on my green team (general surgery), which was more like the fun group of *M.A.S.H* surgeons on TV.

Witnessing vascular surgery was amazing. To watch a surgery team replace somebody's aorta with tubing was incredible—but it made for long surgeries requiring tremendous bladder control. Apparently surgeons have really huge bladders —or perhaps they don't tell the students that they all wear catheters? I never asked.

We had finished one lengthy surgery where my only thoughts were of the quickest route to the nearest bathroom, when the attending said with a chuckle, "Let's take the gall bladder out as well. We're here anyway." It turned out to be a troublesome removal and for another hour I felt my eyeballs flood over and almost passed out. Meanwhile, the surgeons all seemed to be enjoying themselves around the operating table

A few days later I was in the university hospital, smiling, thinking, *I could be a surgeon; it's fun and the work isn't too bad.*

Then I bumped into the blue team.

The behind-my-back grinning student who had taken my place on the blue team looked absolutely shattered; he'd lost weight and was ghostly pale. He tried to smile as I told him about our team going out for lunch and playing basketball on call. He had won the rock-paper-scissor battle, but I had won the war.

However, all good things must end and it was time for me to experience some surgical sub-specialties.

BURN TEAM

WHY WE DON'T TAKE UNNECESSARY ANTIBIOTICS

As part of our surgery sentence, we were allowed to choose between additional time on a General Surgery team or joining a Surgical Sub-specialty team. The Burn ICU service was known to be challenging and exhausting. Medical students took call every other night and the burn team attending physician had one of the toughest reputations in the hospital. Challenging, exhausting, and daunting were not qualities I looked for in my elective rotations.

But then I was *enthusiastically* advised that I would find no better learning for acute care of really sick patients, and might get practice placing "lines," i.e. putting big tubes into the major vessels in patients' necks or groins—procedures usually reserved for interns and residents—*when* I joined the burn team.

That cheerleading decree came from my clinically over-achieving and brilliant medical student girlfriend. I was not made of her same mettle or intelligence; however, surviving weeks on the burn team was a shorter fate than facing a lifetime of her chagrin if I didn't sign up.

Burn team, here I come.

I mentally girded myself for an intense two weeks under the gruff Burn ICU attending. Then I discovered I would also be working with a surgical resident whose reputation was "arrogant" on his better days. "Asshole" was the word most commonly associated with him. He gained this savory reputation during his intern year when he had repeatedly challenged attending physicians, yelled at nurses, and was abusively harsh to medical students. The senior residents had finally put him in his place and he'd been forced to reflect on why he'd received such a verbal beating.

On top of those appealing work conditions, I would also be caring for patients who had been severely burned. Treating paralyzed burn victims with disfiguring scars, infected and festering wounds, and who were breathing on ventilators, intimidated me—it was going to be challenging work.

It's daunting to walk into an ICU. It's a very tight-knit work environment where the team has worked together under intense and bonding battle conditions. They know each other, joke together, speak the same language, and then in strolls a medical student, dressed like a doctor but with little idea what to do other than stand there and wait to be helped.

I showed up for my first morning hoping my nervous trembling would be mistaken for shivering in the winter cold. To my surprise, the resident was not only friendly, but also seemed to treat me with respect. I immediately thought, *it's a ruse to put me off my guard and make me look stupid in front of the attending for being relaxed.*

Are you starting to think that medical students behave like feral animals, constantly looking for food, shelter, and expecting trouble from every encounter?

The resident explained that the burn team intern was absent for at least a week. I swallowed hard. *Did this mean twice the workload for me?*

He looked around the burn unit—a large ICU with patient rooms surrounding the central nurse and physician work area.

He pointed to one side of the unit and said, "You take that half and I'll cover this half. You're their doctor now." And that was that.

The routine of examining patients, writing notes, and rounding with the attending was basically the same as on other rotations. In the ICU, however, every single minute detail was critical — details like figuring out exactly how much fluid had been lost by the patient (whether from fever, urine, diarrhea or skin loss); how much fluid was replaced; and what method was used to replace it. Knowing such things was essential not only to the patient's care, but also to my avoiding being castrated for ineptitude.

We carefully evaluated patients' wounds; their respiratory status on ventilators; X-rays of their lungs; their lengthy medication lists; and vital sign trends. Every detail had to be ready at the tip of your tongue for the arrival of the burn unit's infamous attending. He was a stocky man with a fierce disposition—something out of *Cujo* meets *Henry V* on *ER*. He was also the epitome of excellence when it came to meticulous patient care and dedication to surgery.

The team for rounds included not only the attending, but also the patient's nurses and a host of other people involved with everything from pharmacology to psychosocial care for the patient's family, and people who were apparently hired for no other reason than to laugh at my mistakes.

Once again "rounding" was a chance to quiz the medical student, but with this attending I did not even consider trying to bullshit an answer. "I don't know" were the right words, but such honesty did little to protect my self-esteem from the attending's disappointed raised eyebrow. The ICU would be absolutely silent, apart from respirators mechanically breathing, as he explained why I should know such a crucial bit of information.

Then he would either say, "Well, tell me tomorrow," or he would take out a pen and diagram the answer out before saying, "I'll expect you to read about this by tomorrow." And I would. These were the simple and terrifying tactics of an incredible teacher who seemed to live at the hospital and cared deeply for his patients.

Burn patients were unique. In order to gain admittance to the burn ICU, their injuries had to be quite severe, usually life-threatening; and at the same time, how those life-threatening injuries occurred was often quite ridiculous. Wile E. Coyote wannabes and Darwin Award contestants filled our ICU census.

But ironically the single worst patient we cared for had no thermal burn, but was a victim of medical treatment. The patient, a young woman, once stunningly beautiful, had been prescribed a common antibiotic, amoxicillin, for what sounded like a common head cold. Rather than improving her cold, the gratuitous antibiotic triggered a severe allergic reaction. Her parents tried using homeopathic remedies to reverse the reaction and had placed her in an herbal bath. Then they repeated this treatment for too long—several days too long, apparently.

When I first saw her, she appeared to have been boiled in

hot oil, a result of a potentially fatal adverse drug reaction called TENS, Toxic Epidermal Necrolysis Syndrome. Her skin was bright red, blistered, and oozing. She required a ventilator to breathe and was being pumped full of medicines for infections, sedation, blood pressure, and pain control. Her body had swelled so much from the reaction and the volume of medications that it was impossible to make out any features of what her face might have looked like prior to taking the unnecessary medicine. On the wall, however, was a picture of the entire family—among them, the most striking by far, was this now unrecognizable girl in her twenties.

Made you think twice about giving or taking antibiotics, especially if they were not really needed in the first place for a viral head cold.

This is a tough chapter to write because the patients were in such a bad way and what the doctors were required to do was not easy work; in fact, it was barely palatable at times—and yet humor was still required to get through the day. The humor was not callous at all, far from it. The nurses, physicians, and all who worked with the patients become very personally tangled in the decisions in how to best care for these injured people. I watched that same resident, the one described as an "asshole" the year before, stand hour after hour at his patients' bedsides, late into every night, watching their vitals flashing, to see if the slightest change in the ventilator settings was making a difference.

As mentioned, the Burn Team required taking call every other night, but it was home call, meaning that you stayed at home and were called back to the hospital if anything happened. If nothing happened on your call night, then you had a nice night at home.

I was working with surgeons, however and if nothing

happened on my call night, the resident would cheerfully ask me the next morning, "Since you got some rest last night, do you want me to call you tonight if anything comes in?"

And I would think, *No, I want to go out and have a glass of wine, see my friends, and not lie in bed awake like I did last night waiting for my pager to go off,* as I replied, "Yes, that would be great. Thank you."

The resident was on home call every single night, so I rightfully looked like a bit pathetic if I said no. I would lie awake all over again, waiting for the pager to go off—which it inevitably did. Despite the lack of sleep however, it was exciting to get called because I was actually rushing to take care of an emergency. I hopped in my frozen car and drove up to the hospital at 3 a.m., barely able to see through the iced-over windshield.

Then I sprinted several floors up to the burn unit where the resident would inform me, "The helicopter will be here in an hour, let's get some rest."

We lay in some empty hospital room beds, waiting for the sound of the ICU doors opening, then we'd run back to find our patient, a young entrepreneur whose methamphetamine lab had blown up in his face.

As I scrubbed off his blistered skin, I was actually yelled at by our gruff attending to get more aggressive—so I scrubbed harder. Taking care of burn patients was a tedious and difficult art, even crude in some ways. The burns alone were bad enough; they had the potential to become infected and were a source of massive fluid loss—so the patient had pain, high risk of serious infection, and was likely to become dehydrated with all the secondary complications, not to mention scarring.

The patient's body was also at risk for an inflammatory response, which would cause his or her body to swell dramatically, including swelling the throat shut—so most every patient required rapid intubation to keep their airways open. Due to pain, most patients were paralyzed and anesthetized by drugs, so they needed a ventilator to breathe, anyway. Being paralyzed meant they could not feed themselves, so we inserted tubes for feeding into their stomachs, placed IV lines to administer fluids and drugs, and inserted more lines into their hearts in order to monitor their cardiac status—all of which provided more potential sources of infections.

So now we had to contend with pain, multiple sources of infection, breathing problems and the associated risks of a ventilator (which were enormous), nutrition, hydration, blood pressure (which meant potential complications with kidneys and brain function)—the list went on and on and you can begin to understand why every detail needed to be meticulously scoured over several times a day—the difference being life or death.

On a quick side note, isn't it amazing that your body can regulate all that stuff by itself when it's healthy?

The morning routine started around 5 a.m. or earlier. As usual, we would go in, examine the patients carefully, and record all the above information. Then we'd write all the patient's notes, including an assessment of what needed to be addressed that day: change antibiotics, change fluid volume into body, change IV lines, change ventilator settings, order lab tests, need for skin grafting, etc.

Then the attending arrived and in the most formal presentation yet, we walked around the packed ICU and discussed each patient. To the credit of the attending surgeons, while these were terrifying moments, as long as they saw you working hard and trying to learn what was going on, they would still push, prod, and make fun of you—but all in an instructional way. I sensed this slightly, but it took the resident pulling me aside one day after I had been ceremoniously raked across some burning coals for not knowing how to accurately describe the pressure-volume curve of a patient with acute respiratory distress syndrome (ARDS).

"Just remember, he does that because he likes you and sees you trying," the resident told me. "If he ignores you, that means he doesn't want to waste his time with you." There again was that arrogant resident, taking time to console me with words that got me through the rotation.

After peeling what was left of myself off the floor after rounds, my next task was to start or replace patients' central lines—a procedure that involved sticking a large needle into somebody's groin or neck, feeding long wires into their blood vessel, and then sewing a larger tube into their skin after passing it into the blood vessel. It was actually a risky procedure because you were holding onto long wires that fed into people's large blood vessels, often directly into their heart.

There were horror stories of residents accidentally letting go of the feed wire, and when the loose wire hit the heart tissue, the patient's heart would go into ventricular fibrillation, a possibly deadly code situation. The culpable resident simultaneously experienced a life-threatening heart rhythm. Indeed, heart failure probably would've been a better way to go compared to the death-by-humiliation of recounting the mistake in front of seventy people at the weekly morbidity and mortality conference.

To guard against such accidental deaths, the chief resident would usually oversee interns or junior residents placing these lines. Students did not normally place central lines, but my resident, now *very* cool in my eyes, had said these were my patients and expected me to be responsible for their care. He showed me how to place a line once and after that lesson, he expected me to place the rest myself.

The single most important medical learning credo is, "*See one, do one, teach one.*" It works.

Besides placing lines, the major surgical procedure in the burn unit is skin grafting—this is where things get graphic. If a person had lost their skin (a bit careless to lose the body's largest organ, I suppose) from burns or subsequent infections, the burn team performed skin grafting. A large piece of healthy skin was shaved off one part of the body and then fed through a machine resembling a pasta maker that punched the skin full of holes so that it resembled fishnet stockings, thus enabling the graft to be spread across a space many times its original surface area. This tissue was then placed over the missing area of skin and stapled into place— but not before the wounded area was first shaved down to make it bleed profusely to provide blood supply to the grafted skin. Let your imagination do its worst. That is enough about that subject.

Our duties beyond the ICU included working in the burn clinic to evaluate recovering burn victims. These clinic sessions allowed us to mentally bestow more *"What were you thinking?"* awards, such as for the schoolteacher who observed a fallen power line across a hiking trail and, through some break in logic, decided to move it out of the way in case anybody touched it accidentally. The subsequent electrical shock that jolted through her body, scarring it deeply, had enough power to throw her twenty feet through the air.

There were numerous people in the clinic who had looked for gas leaks with a lighter, well-meaning children who had spilled hot oil or hot soup off the stove trying to cook for themselves, people who had fallen into campfires, and several who had been struck by lightning.

One burn patient I met was especially interesting. He had been rock climbing in a canyon when he was struck by lightning and had fallen forty feet onto solid rock. He'd been brought into the burn-trauma ICU with injuries from the lightning strike along with a broken neck, collapsed lung, and broken ribs, leg, and spine. It was believed that the lightning bolt had stopped his heart, i.e. killed him, but his heart was jolted back to life by the chest-thumping impact of his body slamming onto rocks from forty feet in the air.

In the objective ICU environment there was not a lot of room for spirituality from the medical practitioners; such beliefs and wishes were left to the families.

But in this case the usually stoic bulldog attending had sat incredulous at the patient's bedside and told him, "You need to take a good hard look at what you're supposed to do with your life. Apparently somebody doesn't want you to die just yet."

To wrap up the burn unit: the last I heard of the young girl who had taken antibiotics for a viral head cold and developed TENS was that she had been transferred to another hospital to await a complete lung transplant. The bulldog attending was (and is) still saving lives on a regular basis.

The resident, well, I gave him my cute neighbor's phone number. They both refused to call each other for several weeks until I forced them into it.

Months later, while working in a small mountain clinic in Colorado, I received a phone call wondering if I would be back in time to attend their wedding the following month.

As for me, I was transferred to the orthopedic service.

ORTHOPEDICS IS THE SURGICAL CLUB FOR VERY COOL PEOPLE. I had once considered applying for an orthopedic residency; however, after my pesky head injuries reduced my ability to learn the names of bones, which I assumed was a requirement to operating on them, I accepted that I wouldn't have the grades to apply for orthopedics, one of the most competitive residency fields. These gals and guys were overachievers since they were conceived; usually becoming national champions of one sport or another before taking time to put you back together again.

Remember Eric Heiden? As an encore to winning too many Olympic gold medals, appearing on too many magazine and cereal box covers, he became one of the country's top cyclists, racing in the Tour de France—and *then* became an orthopedic surgeon.

It's that type of club.

Months later, when I applied to residency programs, I spoke with an orthopedic surgeon friend in charge of admitting new orthopedic residents to our university's program. She had been the U.S. National waterskiing champion and was the only woman to ever drive the ski boat for the World Championships. She informed me that her applicant pool that year included several national champions from various sports, an international musical phenomenon, a guy who had single-handedly escaped a plane crash and saved the majority of the casualties, and a woman who had started and operated a hospital clinic in Africa.

Meanwhile, I had been happily coaching a junior development ski team on my days off from medical school, and drinking tequila (not at the same time).

So what do I remember about orthopedics? First, they are the exception to my description of all surgeons thinking they are the smartest doctors in the hospitals. My orthopedic surgeon friends will look at a stethoscope and laugh, telling you they have no idea how to use it. They are true specialists in the arts and crafts of orthopedics and do not want to spend time doing anything else. That said, they're all really smart too. Secondly, they have the all-time best tools, better than Spicoli's dad's ultimate set of tools (If you're lost and I'm dating myself, watch *Fast Times at Ridgemont High*. It's a must-see). Any handyman or Home Depot fan would drool at the shiny saws and drills these doctors play with on a daily basis. Basically it's advanced carpentry with nerves and blood vessels thrown in for plumbing and electricity. The body worked according to most of the same laws used for construction and engineering—structural foundations, plumbing, and filters. They both need electricity or power to make things work. And some people like big pillars on the front façade to announce themselves; a matter of taste.

The orthopedists are also some of the friendliest doctors in the hospital because they are truly doing what they love. I was familiar with the daily routine after my previous surgical rotations: examine post-surgical patients early in the morning, write notes, round with team, "assist" on operations, and evaluate patients in clinic.

I watched surgeries where spines were fused (lots of blood and smoke), joints were replaced (medieval type hammering and sawing of bones), knees were "cleaned" up, and bones put back together – ORIFs (Open Reduction and Internal Fixation) using rods or plates to hold fractured bones together.

To top off the fun, call nights were taken from home. I was called back to the hospital when trauma cases arrived, usually car accident victims. I was able to scrub into the surgery with the on-call trauma doctor and help put shattered bones back inside the body. Repeatedly examining and treating trauma victims with surgeons would prove to be excellent training for my upcoming rotation in rural medicine—as was the clinic work.

Inside the orthopedic clinic I learned to properly evaluate knee and shoulder injuries. Over and over we moved knees and shoulders through a series of motions until they thought I was doing a decent job myself.

You typically hear about athletes suffering ACL and MCL injuries, or about shoulder injuries involving the rotator cuff. I received excellent teaching in pulling and pushing on knees and shoulders, learning to assess if those ligaments and tendons had been stretched or torn. Hold the lower leg and push the lateral aspect of the knee to create Valgus stress (makes the knee into an "L" shape, that's how I remembered Valgus vs. Varus stress) which stresses the medial collateral ligament (MCL); the Lachman test to test ACL integrity: jerking the lower leg forward (that's not a medical term by the way) and hopefully feeling something keeping it from pulling too far away from the body, that's your ACL. I could write an anatomy book for bozos.

Then there's the shoulder assessment. The knee should only move so many directions: typically flexing and extending (back and forth) with only limited motion anywhere else. The shoulder however is the most mobile joint in the body, it goes all sorts of directions: abduction, adduction, flex, extend, rotate, spin, parry, dodge and once you understand where it moves, you need to learn the normal range of motion degrees for each of those movements. My head injured state of miserable recall voluntarily kicked back in during shoulder evaluations and I struggled to keep all the names, directions, degrees of motions in order. I much preferred the simple back and forth moving knee. But again, quite fortuitously, I studied and learned both those exams.

Because then, after months of living on hospital gruel, holding retractors, and scrubbing my hands, it was time for a required rotation of Rural Medicine.

RURAL MEDICINE—TELLURIDE MEDICAL CLINIC

WHERE A SPIDER BITES MY PENIS

After personally petitioning (i.e. shamelessly groveling), I convinced the Telluride Medical Center, a place usually reserved for medical students from the University of Colorado, to take me on for a month-long rotation. So, one frigid November morning, with pale pallor, bloodshot eyes, and feeling generally skewered from several months on surgical rotations, I arrived in the gorgeous mountain town where my friend Dave lived with his family. Dave and his wife were well liked in the small town; they were the real reason I had been invited to spend the month working with the town's doctors.

Telluride is situated in a box canyon 10,000 feet above sea level, with no easy access in or out. Family practice doctors staffed the town's medical clinic, which handled all the medical issues that transpired in a town at altitude, with a lot of bars, a lot of snow, and a lot of poorly balanced tourists hurtling downhill on skis, and stumbling home at night.

The clinic's work hours were essentially nine to five and

allowed for a few ski runs at lunchtime. On top of this friendly schedule was the fact that the medicine was kind of enjoyable. With the closest hospital an hour away in good road conditions, we were tasked — along with taking care of patients — with rapid decision-making about keeping patients at altitude in a clinic with limited medical facilities.

The day's work revolved around people with colds and sore throats, patients brought off the mountain by the ski patrol with broken wrists, damaged knees and shoulders, the occasional car wreck victim, and to end my first day, a large German shepherd whose paw had been run over (he was fine).

On my first morning in this clinic staffed by beautiful mountain people, I was a bit nervous to see how my abilities would stack up to their expectations—they were accustomed to students from Colorado, and I was from Utah. There's a mild regional rivalry between the two mountain states with Colorado typically considered the cool place to live, while Utah was mostly known for bizarre rules regarding alcohol.

As the first patient arrived on a patrol sled, I hoped to make a decent impression for personal reasons, but also felt my adopted state's reputation was in my medically insecure hands.

The ski patrolman removed his hat and goggles and surprised me with a loud greeting and bear-hug; coincidentally it was an old friend from my summers spent river-guiding—which provided a mild assurance to the clinic staff that I might be somewhat normal, despite being from Utah.

My patrol friend explained that the woman in the sled had twisted her knee. I must have felt a confidence boost from his boisterous greeting, because as the clinic doctor started to ask if I knew how to evaluate a knee injury (I almost laughed), I let my months of surgery kick in and did exactly what I had been schooled to do: I introduced myself to the patient and proceeded to complete a competent and thorough history and exam. I quickly gained the trust of the clinic doctors, and just as importantly, that of the staff and ski patrol.

The slippery mountain and roads, along with a recently installed terrain park for skiers and snowboarders to defy gravity, provided a veritable factory of knee, shoulder, wrist and back injuries. After weeks of seeing a steady stream of patients arriving from the terrain park, I eventually had to ask, only half-kidding, if the medical clinic had sponsored its construction. Apparently not.

Fortunately, my recent months on surgical rotations (and especially orthopedics) provided me with the ideal preparation for treating all these injuries. It was as if I had been purposely assigned the exact rotations I needed to help me make a good impression; but now, instead of seeing the patients the next day in a hospital bed, I ran into them on the sidewalk or in a town store.

I'll admit to some mild gratification when tourists approached me on the street and said, "Thank you again doctor."

There was a certain Norman Rockwell small-town charm in asking the checkout girl at the grocery store, "Judy, how's your back feel?"

After a few weeks I was known in town as Doctor John or Dr. Utah. And in small towns, who you know can be key—like the bartenders at a crowded happy hour or the people in charge of hiring medical providers for popular music festivals. Wonderful people whom I got to know and take care of, and in turn, drink and laugh with over the next years.

On the other hand the small town atmosphere occasionally proved awkward; such as when the manager of the popular bakery in town arrived in clinic complaining that his leg hurt after falling down drunk. The accident occurred several nights prior to our meeting. He had already been diagnosed and treated for a twisted ankle, but now his knee was tender.

I was quite proud of myself for remembering that twisting your ankle could potentially cause a spiral fracture in the fibula and break the bone all the way up by your knee—right where he was now tender. An x-ray confirmed he had a broken proximal fibula. I patted myself on the back, put him in a walking boot, and sent him on his way. Nothing awkward yet, but this is where the small town atmosphere backfires.

Since I had correctly diagnosed his leg injury, he decided to return the next day trusting me with a slightly different problem, this time for pain near his rectum.

Oh, joy of joys.

I examined him and discovered, hidden in the cleft of his left buttock, a bright red, inflamed cyst. I could see why he was in pain; it was bulging, pus-filled, clearly infected, and needing to be drained.

I cleaned the area, numbed it with lidocaine, lanced the cyst with a scalpel, and let the foul liquid flow out of the wound before packing it with gauze to prevent it recurring. No problem, typical treatment protocol.

Doctors see a lot of unsavory stuff and we block a lot of it out. That said, I never ate in his bakery ever again.

More small town charm? Later the following spring, I sat in a sushi restaurant on a first date with a local woman. I looked around the restaurant, smiling at friendly faces, waving to people at the bar, seeing some guy that looked vaguely familiar… I couldn't quite place him, but he looked so familiar. Then I realized I had been doing a testicular exam on him two hours prior. Not quite an appetizing memory at a sushi restaurant—

or anywhere else for that matter. Small town medicine had its merits and drawbacks.

My single best medical school moment also occurred in town that month, the moment that eventually convinced me to go into family practice medicine.

A nine-year-old girl was brought into the clinic on her birthday; she had slipped on ice and bonked her head. She was fine, apart from a few small scrapes that I carefully washed and bandaged. The next day, standing in line at the bakery (pre-cyst draining), I felt an arm wrap around my waist. I looked down to see the same small girl, with her bandaged scrapes, smiling up at me. She turned to her young crowd of friends, arm still around me, and proudly announced, "This is my doctor...and he's the best doctor in the world."

That was it—I was hooked.

Medical students are pretty beaten down and the ego boost from being called "doctor" by a nine-year-old might have the makings of several paragraphs in a psychology book, but for the moment, it felt nicer than being humiliated in an operating room for not remembering the name of the doctor involved in the land-breaking Japanese study proving that CT scans were more sensitive in revealing appendicitis than ultrasounds.

The clinic work itself was what I had imagined practicing medicine would be about in the first place: taking care of sick and injured people in a remote location. The doctors enjoyed their work and in turn were fun to work with and very instructional. I kept hearing about one doctor, in particular, who had become a guru in the world of expedition and wilderness medicine—he had even been hired by NASA to help with medicine on the space shuttle. "Howard" (Hodo) worked on weekends and I was really excited to finally work with him my first weekend on call.

I was staying with my friend Dave in his mountain house, where I slept in the third floor loft. The night before I was scheduled to work with Hodo, I climbed up the ladder to the loft, promptly fell asleep and then, suddenly, was jolted awake by a sharp pain in my crotch.

I immediately sat upright and proceeded to smack my head on the loft ceiling; then I reached down to turn on the light and saw bite marks on my penis. Two fang marks. The double fang marks of a spider on my penis. My penis! Holy mother of merde crap and shit!

I frantically searched for the culpable beast under the many blankets, but couldn't locate him, although I knew there were many spiders in the loft.

I tried working my paltry medical knowledge into a rational thought process despite a voice in my head shouting, "DIAL 911! DIAL 911!"

OK, think...Spider bites, two to be worried about. First, black widows. Their bite causes pain at the bite location, swelling, flu symptoms, and abdominal pain.

My stomach hurt, but I couldn't tell if that was from the bite or from the thought of losing my penis. So I couldn't rule out the black widow.

Second, brown recluse spiders—they're found in dark corners of houses, like basements and lofts. Lofts. Shit! Their bite causes necrosis and ulceration at the bite mark. DOUBLE SHIT!

I began having severe abdominal pain and ran downstairs to look at the bite in better light. The two red marks were definitely there and I decided to peruse my friend's bookshelves for any medical texts. Of course Dave had no medical texts in the house and there was no way I was going to wake him or his wife to show them the bite mark on my penis. And remember, this was pre-Google and there were no Internet medical chat rooms to discuss genital spider bites.

I thought about calling the clinic. From what I could recall, as I hyperventilated in the thin mountain air, there was nothing to do for either type of spider bite. So the thought of getting one of my bosses out of bed at 2:30 in the morning to glance at my penis and say there was nothing to do was far from appealing. So I waited to see what symptoms arose.

Lying back in the loft after one more futile effort to locate the culprit, I attempted to sleep.

When you think your penis is going to become necrotic and fall off, it's not possible to sleep. And when you're convinced your penis is going to fall off and you can't sleep, you get to lie awake pondering your chances of ever having sex again...Not very good!

So I ran downstairs to look at the bite mark one more time —no change. I tromped back upstairs, climbed the ladder to the loft, and tried sleeping again—when suddenly a new concern seized my already strung-out synapses. What if the bite venom is neuro-toxic? *What if I survived the bite but could never get an erection?* I decided that I better check if the nerves were working, and was relieved to find that I was currently able to attain an erection—a good start.

I next debated whether putting ice on my penis to slow the poison was a good idea. For the sake of my penis having a fighting chance, I tried it for several minutes. Not enjoyable.

Finally by 6 a.m., having checked the bite site and my erection ability 243 more times, I decided I was going to live. The lack of acute symptoms thus far made it unlikely my attacker was a black widow, which left the brown recluse, and that meant I needed to look up any medical treatments available to avoid necrotic penis ulcerations.

It was far from appealing to meet the hip and suave, cool doctor in town with the greeting, "Hi, nice to meet you. Want to check out a bite on my penis?" Instead I drove down to the clinic early enough to read up on spider bites before anyone else arrived, but there was nothing really helpful in the medical books either.

I decided I would check on my penis every ten minutes throughout the day to see if there were any signs of it falling off or having giant ulcerations. Not much of a plan and Hodo would likely think I had some sort of bladder control issue.

When I did meet Howard he turned out to be a very laidback, movie star-looking guy with a super cool demeanor. He switched gears when emergencies arrived and ran the show with confidence and efficiency. Which was good, because the day ahead of us would set a record for the number of patients seen in the town clinic. The day became so busy that I forgot to do my periodic ten-minute penis checks. Suddenly we had a clinic filled with patients in every room, lying on every trauma bed, sitting on every stretcher in the hall, and lining up in the waiting area.

At some point as we ran from room to room, Howard, who had quickly gained confidence in my medical abilities, pulled me aside, looked me in the eye and said, "Right now what we need is for you to be a doctor. Go take care of those three rooms and tell them you're a doctor. Can you do that?"

With that vote of confidence I went into the rooms, sewed up a laceration on a woman's face, diagnosed a torn ACL, and managed a car accident victim. This was now my new favorite moment in medicine.

Sometime later that night, after seeing seventy-six patients and laughing a lot, it was time for us to head out. Dave had told me to meet him at a nearby holiday party.

One block later I was in a house, consuming gin and tonic after gin and tonic, talking with a lot of attractive women and realizing I was drunk. But I had a plan—I would just walk back and sleep in the clinic; that way I could wake up, enjoy coffee and breakfast, and already be at work in the morning. I went back to the clinic, lay down on the couch, and slept.

The plan proceeded perfectly until 5 a.m.

At 5 a.m. I heard the clinic door open. My eyes focused hazily on Howard standing over me, "Oh good, you're here," he said, "A kid with a seizure is coming in."

I could barely see and was probably legally drunk. Several seconds later the ambulance pulled up and there we were, hovering over a twelve-year-old boy who had apparently looked like he was having a seizure but now looked absolutely fine.

I was supposed to examine him but all I could think, besides wishing the percussion player inside my skull would stop, was that I was going to give the kid another seizure when I breathed near him. Eventually we decided to send him to a hospital just to be safe—which would thankfully give me time to get coffee and wake up.

Before seizure boy was out the door, however, I heard another patient in the trauma room. I wandered in the direction of what sounded like a roman vomitorium. There, waiting for me, was a drunken patient, violently retching blood and bile into a basin.

Hungover and hanging out with a vomiting drunk who smelled worse than me was a poor way to start my Sunday. I was still supposed to be sleeping before going out for a relaxing cup of coffee. Instead I, the idiot who had drunk one too many drinks, was telling this wretched-smelling fellow that it was probably a bad idea to drink so much if it made him vomit blood.

As more and more patients decided to spend their Sunday morning checking into the clinic, my relaxing coffee moment became a pipedream. The clinic became a blur as I struggled to deal with the combination of a whopping hangover, and patients with more serious problems, like a lack of common sense.

One elderly woman was very concerned that she had become short of breath ever since arriving in town and maybe had a little cough and fever too. From her description I was worried she had pneumonia and ordered a chest x-ray.

As we waited for the X-ray I asked her some more questions, including, "Have you ever had a cough like this before?"

"Oh yes," she replied, "I have a cough like this all the time."

"Really? You should probably see a doctor for it."

"I see several doctors for it," she told me, "I have some lung disease I can't pronounce. It's because I smoked three packs of cigarettes a day for thirty years."

"So have you been short of breath like this before?"

"Oh yes, all the time."

"What do you mean all the time?"

"Well, at home in Texas, if I don't wear my oxygen, like the doctors tell me, I usually pass out."

Texas, for the geographically challenged, is at sea level. And this lovely woman was currently wasting her already diminished breath, along with what few of my brain cells were working, on concerns about why she was short of breath at an altitude of 10,000 feet while not wearing her required oxygen. I should have sent her out to buy me coffee after making her write, "I will wear my oxygen" five hundred times on the chalkboard.

One of the beautiful things about working in medicine at 10,000 feet was that only moderately healthy people could survive there comfortably. None of the chronically sick hospital patients with the volumes of medical problems I was used to examining even existed at this altitude. Most patients we encountered were acutely sick or injured, did not like going to the doctor, and genuinely wanted to get better—after months working in the hospital setting, I thought this was a revolutionary mindset.

For example, the next guy I took care of that morning was an otherwise healthy young man visiting Telluride for his wedding. He and his fiancée were to be married the next day. The poor guy arrived in our clinic after having fevers all night along with coughing, a sore throat, and an achy body. He was now vomiting, and looked really sick; influenza-flu type sick.

After taking down his medical history, I examined him and noted some mild nasal congestion, but everything else appeared normal. We treated him for a bad cold combined with mild altitude sickness and told him to take several ibuprofen for his fevers. Hopefully he would be feeling better for his wedding the next day. It felt good to take care of sick people who had the desire to recover.

The rest of the day passed in much the expected fashion, with me tired, hungry and looking forward to going to sleep that night. Then I received a phone call. It was the sick fiancé from the morning. He was calling back, which usually meant something was wrong. I was already worried about him, worried that perhaps he had early signs of pneumonia that I had missed.

I answered the phone, "Hello, this is John, what's going on?"

"Hi doc, I'm not doing well at all and you said to call if I got worse."

That was how you were trained to cover your ass in medicine, by telling people to call or come back immediately if anything got worse and documenting that you had done so. I just hoped patients had the decorum not to take me up on such generous offers.

"Tell me what's going on," I replied.

"Well, I still feel sick and you told me to take some ibuprofen."

"Right."

"Well I took them and now my stomach hurts, a lot."

Shit. In my hung-over state I couldn't remember if I had asked him about any problems with stomach ulcers and now I had probably caused him to have a life-threatening stomach bleed. So I asked him if he had any stomach problems already.

"No, my stomach is fine normally," he told me.

I breathed a sigh of relief and asked, "How many ibuprofen did you take?"

"Sixteen."

"Say again?"

"Sixteen."

"Sorry, did you say *sixteen?*"

I swallowed back my sigh of relief and tried to recall if I had told him to take sixteen ibuprofen pills. Not likely.

"And now your stomach hurts?" I asked.

"Yeah, a real lot, real bad, I can't stand it."

Well if he wasn't sick before, it sounded like I had made him sick now. I told him to get back to the clinic so we could re-evaluate him. I was now convinced he had a massive GI bleed from ibuprofen eating into his gut. Probably my fault and I would be heading for a lawsuit and losing my license before I even had one. *But who the hell goes and takes sixteen-ibuprofen?*

When he and his concerned fiancée arrived back at the

clinic, I decided to have Howard accompany me for the whole talk. We discussed exactly what he was experiencing and finally Howard asked if maybe they should call the priest and cancel the wedding since the illness seemed to be worsening.

Since the patient was probably going to die from a stomach bleed, I thought the least of his concerns should be whether or not to cancel the priest—*actually, keep the priest; we're going to need him for a different ceremony.*

Howard and I stepped outside the room to discuss what to do. He asked me exactly how the patient had presented that morning to make sure we were not missing some serious diagnosis. Then we headed back into the room, but not before Howard told me that he thought the guy was kind of weird. Howard sat down and told the affianced couple that maybe they should cancel the wedding plans until the flu resolved.

"Really, you think so?" the guy asked. As Howard confirmed his belief that it was best to cancel the wedding plans, I saw the patient repress a smile of relief. He bounded out of the clinic, practically skipping, feeling fine.

This guy had been so put out by his impending nuptials that he had literally made himself sick. Like I said, now biting my tongue, healthy normal people who only came in when they were really sick and wanted to get better—in this ibuprofen popping, nutjob's case, by having his wedding called off. No problem. Totally normal behavior.

And let me comment how that was intelligent medicine by Howard. In between treating fractured bones, car accident victims, and their bleeding spleens, he was taking care of the psychosocial needs of conjugally reluctant tourists. Finally the day ended and we sat and laughed about surviving another crazy day together.

Later that night I headed back to Dave's house, where he

was waiting with a beer for me to recap the day's nonsense. And soon afterwards I was peacefully asleep after a long, entertaining forty-eight hours.

But suddenly I was jerked awake by the same sharp pain on my penis. I had forgotten about the spider and this bite felt just like the first one. I tore the covers off, committed to exposing the fanged rascal who had assaulted me for the last time. No such luck, it escaped again.

I lay back down and as I rolled over felt the pain yet again.

And then I realized that I was lying on the culprit. My watchband. My Velcro watchband lay crushed beneath me. Those fang marks, the ones that had kept me up all night, vigilantly perusing my penis and checking its erectile function, were not fang marks at all; just the Velcro on my watchband pinching me as I rolled over in my sleep.

I haven't worn a watch since.

INTERNAL MEDICINE

NOBODY EXPECTS THE HOSPITAL
INQUISITION

I returned to Salt Lake City for my next rotation, Internal Medicine ("medicine") - treating adult patients sick enough to be admitted to the hospital. Show up early, examine patients, write notes, round on patients, etc.; we knew the routine, the language, the required work, and were now expected to be productive team members.

It looked like it would be a strait forward rotation. But that's just not how life works. We now interrupt this medical journal to comment on human emotions and relationships, all of which weighed heavily upon these six weeks of medicine.

During the past months I had yet to truly grieve the death of my friend John. After his accident, I had worked in-patient rotations requiring long hours, weekends and call-nights in the hospital. As a result of working non-stop, I had been able to remain emotionally walled off. But then my time in Telluride served up an elixir of humanity. I had slept, eaten meals at a table, made new friends, been treated like a human being, and even had a few days off. That healthy prescription of civilized living was a tonic for those icy protective walls; unbeknownst to me, a slow melt began which resulted in the barricades surrounding my emotions releasing a deluge of heartache. Out of nowhere, waves of grief pummeled me. For weeks afterwards, as I started my new medicine rotation, the after-shocks left me blubbering and unbalanced.

I tell you about my mental state because: 1) my memories of this rotation are clouded by a combination of emotional instability and several other challenging events. 2) I'll use that emotional breakdown to remind all of you, when seeing your medical providers, that they are people too. Some days, events outside our control make it hard to be our absolute best, no matter how hard we try, and sometimes all you can muster is to survive the day. So, be kind.

Back to Medicine: After my time enjoying rural outpatient medicine, I was brought back to the reality of hospital life by a zealous nutcase pixie of a chief resident who *loved* medicine. As in, she loved medicine so much she wanted to marry it; she breathed and danced, medicine, waved a glittery, magical medicine wand, and I don't even think she existed in the real world outside the hospital…truthfully, I'd never seen her before or since. She was an avatar of what the residency wanted me to become. She expected me to diligently read several textbooks and journals on every single patient case, to visit sick patients who weren't even on our team, and to constantly engage in cheerful discussions about medicine.

I wanted to hold these expectations against her, as there was never enough time to finish our own assigned work, let alone find journal articles to review; but I couldn't, she was so enthusiastic, so downright giddy, sitting with me and reading all the material herself, anything she could find on each patient case, she scoured over and shared with me. While she was poring over a patient's chart on our first night together, fascinated by some relatively normal blood test values, and I was trying to keep my eyes open, I was paged to go admit a new patient.

The patient turned out to be a very nice, previously healthy, farmer from Idaho, complete with worn flannel shirt and dusty overalls. His sons had brought him to the hospital because he had been coughing up blood for several days. Coughing up blood was not usually a sign of good health; so he had a lot of X-rays and blood tests done to see if he had pneumonia. The X-rays did not appear normal and his fever kept increasing, so the ER admitted him to our service where we ordered a CT scan.

Later that night his chest CT revealed multiple large pockets of infection throughout both of his lungs. This was not a normal finding either and needed some investigation. Eventually an echocardiogram (an ultrasound of his heart) helped diagnose him with isolated tricuspid valve endocarditis; that was believed to be the source of the infection in his lungs.

Each of the four chambers of your heart has a valve that, when healthy, allows blood to pump out and not flow backwards. The tricuspid valve allows blood to flow from the heart's right atrium into the right ventricle, which pumps the blood into the lungs to pick up oxygen. As blood pumped through this patient's heart, the bacteria chewing up his tricuspid heart valve jumped into the bloodstream and was pumped into his pulmonary blood vessels, showering bacteria throughout his lung tissue.

Medically it was interesting because we could not find any cases of isolated tricuspid valve endocarditis in healthy people. (Side note: you never want to be the "interesting" medical case.) Usually these infections were found in immunocompromised patients, such as people who had AIDS, or perhaps in IV drug users. So my chief resident could barely control her enthusiasm; she had discovered a medical pot of gold at the end of an infected rainbow.

It was left to me to perform a very thorough history and physical exam because it was critical to figure out where this infection had originated. I was now forced to re-visit the patient and repeatedly ask this hardworking, salt-of-the-earth farmer, in front of his grown sons, if he was using recreational IV drugs or having a homosexual affair—both of which he denied. I tried waiting until his sons were looking away and asked him again if he was certain he had not injected drugs or had a homosexual affair…and again he denied either action.

I reported his denials to my chief resident. She decided he must be lying and told me to go back and force a confession.

I went back to the farmer's room and asked again if he was certain he had never abused IV drugs or been involved with anyone in a homosexual relationship? He flatly repeated his denials of either case and I returned to the resident with his answers.

Instead of believing me, she was convinced he was hiding part of his Idaho farm life from his family. We stormed back to his room together and asked the family to leave. Then she demanded he come clean; had he been shooting up drugs or sleeping with other men? And again he denied it all. At this point I was feeling rather embarrassed for this polite man with a sky-high fever, dripping sweat and being ruthlessly interrogated.

The resident and I reported his denials to the attending physician.

Minutes later the attending, resident, and I were back in the room with the family. This time the attending physician asked him to please just be honest and tell us if he had been injecting drugs or involved in homosexual relationships on the farm.

The poor guy had a 103-degree fever, was hacking up blood, and doing his best to politely tolerate an inquisition from us regarding his social behavior when all he wanted was to get better. I was waiting for lie detectors, thumbscrews, and interrogation lamps to arrive.

My resident, she of the extensively-research-the-ailments-of-every-patient-in-Utah, was beyond delighted by this case of isolated tricuspid valve endocarditis in a previously healthy patient, and gleefully made me do literary searches all night for any similar cases while she danced merry jigs with visions of speaking tours and awards on the AMA circuit. She then recommended that I write up the case for publishing; an idea that sounded fun for zero seconds whatsoever.

On day two of our patient's Spanish Inquisition themed hospital stay, we repeated his physical exam and noticed a tiny pustule on his elbow that blended into all the other farm induced scrapes and scratches on his arms. He remembered he had torn his shirt on an old fence a week or two ago that caused a small cut. The bacteria from the scratch matched the bacteria in his lungs. Huh. It was decided that his elbow scratch was the source of the infection – no publishing tours and no lurid tales of drug fueled raves on the farms of Idaho.

SOCIALLY THINGS BECAME MORE INTERESTING FOR ME, AS WELL. One of the girls I had innocently flirted with at the party in Telluride—the gin and tonic night where I thought myself witty and slept alone in the clinic—well she wrote me a letter which arrived home while I was on call. My girlfriend, the same strait-A-student with whom I had been living for almost two years, decided it looked like an important letter to open and read herself. I promptly received a phone call wondering why a woman in Telluride was writing to say she was sick and the only cure might be to see Dr. Utah.

Hmmm...No real social protocol to fall back on here. The letter did not go over well and I asked my resident if I could run home for an emergency. I was emotionally not handling anything properly and will admit this new stressor along with lack of sleep did not result in me managing the letter situation admirably; flippantly explaining the girl probably was sick and just asking for medical advice.

The relationship eventually culminated in my girlfriend presenting the ultimatum that I choose between her or my going back to the Telluride Medical Clinic in March.

Her insecurity regarding the letter, however innocent the vein in which it had been written, was understandable. I was the idiot who had drunkenly flirted at a party. I naively believed that my girlfriend of all people, given her dedication to medicine, would understand my desire to return to Colorado to further my positive medical experience, and be able to look past a one-night affair of words. Apparently not.

Telluride was beautiful in March and our relationship had been on the rocks for months—which I admit didn't excuse my flirting. But that was the end of that. She left for a weekend and expected me to be gone when she returned.

Don't feel badly for her; she's brilliant, funny, and beautiful, and several months later she met somebody way smarter than me who was training to be an orthopedic surgeon. Weeks later she called to gloat that they were happily engaged after he piloted a helicopter out to a boat that he then captained to some iceberg in order to propose. I told you orthopedic doctors are overachievers. So they got married and the marriage didn't last. For those of you concerned, she's happily remarried with beautiful children and works as a high-powered radiologist at a fancy hospital in some lovely town.

Medical Heroes

I'M GOING TO SHARE A STORY THAT OCCURRED DURING THAT SAME month because it defines the level of dedication, selflessness and heroism that exists in the world of medicine. First, I'll re-introduce you to one of the characters in the story: One year earlier, for the now ex-girlfriend's birthday, I had arranged a surprise party. Her birthday was a mild point of contention as she was born exactly one week before me, a fact she brought up frequently during arguments, informing me that she would never date a younger man ever again. (Please note: she was putting me on alert early on that she planned to move on.) I admit I wasn't altogether mature in our relationship, either; once, during an argument, she asked what I would do if anything happened to her, I spontaneously started singing, "Ding-dong, the witch is dead!" To her credit, she laughed.

Back to the surprise: As we drove to a restaurant in the mountains where friends were waiting, we encountered a long line of traffic and were diverted off the freeway. I became anxious that the traffic would interfere with the birthday surprise—but we made it up the canyon, the surprise worked and we enjoyed a fun party.

Do you remember the air-med nurse from my pre-med school days, the flight nurse who was starting med school? The one who calmed down a violent patient with the line, "You can either pee in this cup or I'm going to stick this big tube in your dick. What do you want to do?" We were waiting for that guy to show up—and he finally saunters into the restaurant, back-lit as usual, his hair blowing in the unseen breeze that followed him everywhere, with his clothes splattered in blood.

Turns out that the reason we had been directed off the highway was because a car had jumped the median and struck another car head on causing all sorts of trauma. There were multiple unconscious victims. Our friend Steve had been driving right behind the car that was struck. He jumped out and was able to open several people's collapsed airways, do a tracheotomy (cut a hole in their neck to let in air), call in and direct helicopters to land on the freeway, etc. He saved three, maybe four lives, and still showed up at the party, ready for a tequila. These life-saving heroic moments happened to Steve so frequently that I was convinced he was some guardian angel-type hero.

As a medical student Steve had continued to fly for Air-Med. One winter day, while I was on that emotionally laden month of internal medicine, Steve was flying with his team and saving lives as usual, with his wife only days away from delivering their first child.

There had been a backcountry ski accident high in the mountains involving a young couple. The husband had fallen and broken both femurs. He was going to die if he wasn't evacuated. But there was a major problem preventing the evacuation, a violent storm was pounding the mountains, closing the roads, and leaving almost no visibility. They tried a helicopter rescue right away in the early evening, but had been forced to turn back because of the blizzard.

When I entered the hospital the following morning, I could feel a dark, palpable mood weighing down the hospital air. In the cafeteria I overheard two doctors talking about an accident involving Air-Med.

The Air-Med team had been faced with the dilemma of staying grounded due to the terrible flying conditions, but knowing that the snowboarder was going to die if they didn't pick him up.

They were heavily advised not to fly.

With a person's life at stake, not a single person on the team hesitated, they all voted to go back up again.

The team flew back into the mountains, back into the raging storm one more time. And they succeeded; they made it up the canyon and loaded the injured man onboard. They took off, flying into fierce, gusting winds and disappeared under heavy snowfall and darkness, heading back to the waiting hospital.

Then a blast of wind slammed the helicopter into the mountain cliffs. Everybody onboard was killed, pilot, nurses, and patient.

I was hit by a terrible realization. I called Steve's wife, herself the waterskiing national champion orthopedic surgeon. Steve had been scheduled to fly that night and had gone up on the earlier attempt that had turned back. As fate would have it, ten minutes before the fatal rescue attempt, another young flight nurse, Ryan, asked to switch flights with Steve and had gone up instead. The night before the accident, Ryan's wife had surprised him with the news that she was pregnant with their fourth child.

Hundreds of flight crews from around the country, friends, people whose lives had been saved by Air-Med, all came to pay respects, mourn, and support all those devastated by the loss.

Steve's wife gave birth a few days later, and they named their son Ryan, after the brave flight nurse who flew that night instead of him.

INPATIENT PEDIATRICS & RSV

AS THOUGH TO BREATHE WERE LIFE!
(ULYSSES—TENNYSON)

My next rotation was Inpatient Pediatrics, caring for patients admitted to the children's hospital. Being in a new hospital meant facing new nurses, new places where they hid charts, new computer systems with new codes and new passes just to get into the patient wards.

The pass cards at the children's hospital were all coded to the precise date and minute when we were rotating through a pediatric service, which would one day prove quite awkward as my access to patient wards ended at midnight on a night I was on call; didn't turn into a pumpkin, but was trapped, alone, at 12:01 am, in between doors needing an access card. Apart from these differences the work was much the same as being on the adult inpatient hospital team: rounds, charts, lectures, eat when you can, etc.

Fortunately everyone generally liked working at the children's hospital. First of all, the cafeteria meals resembled real food, at least compared to the University's cafeteria. Next, pediatric doctors and nurses are overwhelmingly friendly; you have to be a really nice person to dedicate your life to caring for kids. Third, the resident lounge was continually re-stocked with cookies and snacks on such a regular basis that I considered applying to the pediatric residency program based on the economics of free food access alone.

Then, one morning, during rounds, I had a terrible fever and felt completely nauseated. It was on this fateful morning that we were supposed to taste all the different pediatric medicines typically prescribed to kids so we could be empathetic doctors when we prescribed antibiotics and cough medicines to small fussy eaters (this idea sounds horrible all these years later).

The chief resident kept forcing me to swallow the horrible-smelling liquids, as if I was a sick kid and didn't know what was good for me. I finally did vomit and was sent home from school. It's possible that my healthy indulgence in the cookie tray triggered the stomach bug more than being force-fed syrupy pediatric medicines; but regardless the cause, the vomiting temporarily curbed any pediatric aspirations.

Children's hospitals during the winter months are war zones. Patient beds overflow, families live in hallways, helicopters fly all day and night, and everybody helps out by working extra shifts with their eyelids sagging. Working as a resident in the children's hospital several years later, my pager alert buzzed so frequently that the batteries wore out every 48-hours. Winter was the season where almost every single person under two years of age picked up a respiratory infection and filled the hospital beyond capacity. The major scourge of the season was RSV.

Respiratory Syncytial Virus (RSV) season fills the hospital quickly, so you want to book rooms early. RSV is a common virus that infects infants and toddlers, triggering cold symptoms in some kids and bronchiolitis in others. Children with the latter have a hard time breathing due to inflammation in their smaller airways. Younger kids with RSV bronchiolitis develop wheezing from the inflammation, which can then trigger respiratory distress. When those small kids are forced to breathe hard and fast, they use accessory breathing muscles (muscles not typically used to breathe when you're relaxed).

If you've ever seen a kid or athlete inhaling so forcefully that their ribs poke out or neck muscles bulge, those are accessory breathing muscles. When those muscles are overused, they can actually wear out. Once a kid exhausts accessory muscles, they've run out of energy to breathe; they've literally worn out their breathing muscles. At that point they are in respiratory failure and there's nothing you can do at home. Those kids need respiratory support immediately or they die—which is what kept the helicopters busy flying day and night with nurses emergently treating kids in respiratory distress and failure while they attempted get back to the hospital in time to save their lives.

My entire existence on the in-patient pediatric service was consumed with admitting and discharging little runny-nosed patients with RSV. Every day our team would discharge thirty-four kids and admit another thirty-six, all with RSV. I'm not sure I actually laid eyes on half the kids. I wrote the same admitting notes and orders over and over and over and in between, wrote discharge notes and orders over and over and over. That was the entire hazy, sleepless month: write identical notes, hear wheezing, wash hands, order breathing treatments and oxygen, confirm positive RSV test, write admit note, write discharge note...until finally the month ended and I caught my breath and some sleep.

Medical students were not only overwhelmed by the sheer

volume of the workload, but also forced to deal with a whole new scale of medicine, as the patients were much smaller. Apart from the obvious difference in clothing sizes, pediatric patient care also required everything to be measured in metric doses. Everything you did to a child in the hospital, whether giving IV fluids, injecting medicine doses, or offering corn flakes, was calculated in "milligrams per kilogram per day per dose," mg/kg, pronounced "migs per kig." So there were multiple areas to screw up small numbers on a large scale.

We'll return to the children's hospital for lots of pediatric work and pediatric stories during the residency years. So for now, let's jump ahead to my return to the Telluride Medical Clinic.

A Return to the Telluride Mountain Clinic

SEVERAL HOURS AFTER FINISHING THE LASHING OF INPATIENT pediatrics during RSV season, I returned to the Telluride Medical Center, where two other medical students were also working that month. These students admitted they had been nervous to meet me as my reputation from my previous months in the clinic was pretty stellar, and they worried I would make them look bad. Which I thought a ridiculous idea as I was still consumed by my head-injured lack of medical confidence.

Since this is a short chapter, let me discuss the imposter syndrome I suffered as a future, and now current, doctor. You might have noticed a bit of a paradox in that I believe myself more or less medically incompetent, while receiving high marks and taking good care of my patients.

Perhaps a lot of people, in various work arenas feel this way in life, a sense of, "Who am I to do this work?" *What do I know? Won't they see right through me and realize I'm terrified? That I don't know what I'm doing? Everyone else looks like they know what they're doing. I feel like I'm just playing doctor. They're going to take my license away any day now.*

That was my inner monologue every time I would casually ask a patient, "So, how long have you had this sore throat?" Imposter syndrome is a colossal waste of energy.

I legitimately had an inferiority complex about what I might have missed, along with my short-term memory, during the first year of medical school. Additionally, my ability to retain facts, while improved, had never fully recovered. I did however possess a few good qualities for eventually becoming a doctor. Most importantly, I was good at listening.

Future medical people take this message to heart: Listen to your patients. They know themselves better than you ever will. And parents know their children better than you ever will. My own corollary to that rule is: pay close attention when a patient returns and says something is still not right or that the doctor they saw previously did not listen to them; I swear, nine times out of ten, it saved my ass and the patient's health, to acknowledge and respond to the fact that they knew something had been missed.

To my school's credit, we had been instructed that the number one reason people take legal action against a doctor is not because something went wrong, it's that the patient did not feel the medical provider listened to them. Even if something went medically askew, if the patient felt the doctor had listened and acted appropriately, they were unlikely to pursue legal action.

In over twenty years of practice, I have never been sued. I

sat through one deposition involving a patient who died after being seen in the ER and treated in the hospital. I had seen the patient beforehand and fortunately had very clear notes documenting that I recommended the patient go to the ER for immediate evaluation and treatment. It just ended up being an unfortunate case of a young man who died a few days later in the hospital.

Other positive doctor qualities: I worked hard and I had no ego preventing me from admitting I did not know something. In uncertain situations, I was willing to take time to look up the proper treatment or call someone who could direct me appropriately. I think patients appreciated that I cared about their health enough to fall behind in my schedule—although there were certainly times I wondered if I cared more about the patient's health than they did themselves, as they described nightly routines of couch-surfing with a feed-bucket of fast-food.

Regardless, I was back in Telluride where people generally took care of themselves—well, at least before happy hour.

The clinic's medical director was a compassionate doctor who took thorough care of her patients and ran the clinic well. She expected medical students to write articles about health for the local newspaper and assigned us medical chores, like calling patients with their lab results. I realize that these were reasonable requests, given her role was to teach us how to be good doctors. But her thoroughness and reasonable expectations drove me crazy.

Despite her efforts to derail my fun month with medical teaching and appropriate requirements, I managed to enjoy springtime in the ski town environment and once again, worked with Howard. As usual he attracted the most exciting clinic days—maybe because he only worked weekends.

One Saturday, busy with a stream of patients arriving by ambulance, sled dog, on foot, or riding moose, a high school freshman was brought off the mountain in a ski patrol sled. She was on a school ski trip and had crashed into a forest of trees. Crashing into trees was generally traumatic. After the initial evaluation to clear her neck and back of serious injuries, Howard went to see more patients while I completed her physical exam.

She was certainly a little bruised, but overall seemed OK—until I pushed on her left upper abdomen, which evoked some mild tenderness. I pushed again, wanting to re-check and make sure I wasn't imagining her discomfort. Sure enough, every time I pressed on her left upper abdomen, she squirmed and said it hurt. Her repeated tenderness made me nervous because after trauma, pain in the left upper abdomen can be a sign of a ruptured spleen and people can bleed to death from ruptured spleens.

I pushed one more time, explaining that it never feels good to have someone jam their hand deep into your belly. This time the pain made her jump and I decided it was time to call for Howard to take a look.

When Howard examined her abdomen, and she once again jumped when he pushed in that pesky left upper quadrant, he promptly agreed her abdomen was tender and that my concern was justified.

Why would I not just believe her that her abdomen hurt and send her by jet to the closest hospital?

Well, that's an expensive decision. It's not easy as a medical student to be certain about what's real, what's normal, and what's genuinely concerning with every patient you evaluate. Translating book learning to feeling comfortable with physical exams takes time and requires seeing the real thing repeatedly.

There were only so many times, however, that you could be present to examine someone with a traumatically ruptured spleen. And there were not a lot of volunteers willing to rupture their spleen so we could practice palpating their wounded belly.

Additionally, the cost of labs and radiology studies could be quite traumatic to a patient's financial wellbeing, so you did not send every patient with a tender belly to the emergency room for a CT scan. You tried to be judicious with who needed additional exams or who to send away by ambulance or jet. I actually felt guilty when I sent patients for an MRI or X-ray and nothing showed up as abnormal. I wanted to apologize to those patients for the trouble I had put them through. But in that small clinic, the problem was that besides pushing on her belly and giving her IV fluids, there was very little we could do for her to evaluate or treat a ruptured spleen—and even sending for a helicopter or fixed wing (both very expensive) to get her to the hospital would still take an hour.

Howard decided we could observe her for a short time, make sure she was stable, and then send her away by ambulance. We checked her blood pressure repeatedly to make sure it wasn't plummeting—a sign that she was losing blood internally. Howard then told me to start a big IV line, "…just in case."

Just in case meant, in case she hemorrhaged blood due to a ruptured spleen and we needed to keep her alive by pumping her full of IV fluids until she could be flown to a hospital for surgery.

While Howard monitored the girl and her vital signs, I went to take care of the backlog of patients with typical coughs and colds… and then the ski patrol arrived with another high school student who had crashed skiing. This patient had careened past the spleen bruising forest and had instead chosen to smash into a log fence with his low back.

The first thing he told me was that I should call his dad immediately because his dad was a neurosurgeon. The idea of calling a neurosurgeon to discuss his son's spine injury and neurological status was as appealing to me as calling NASA with some ideas for how to build a really fast space ship.

Talking with real doctors when they were your patients was horrible. As a medical student you felt that everything coming out of your mouth sounded stupid to a real doctor. I remembered all too vividly asking basic questions of patients in hospital beds, and when they informed me that they were a doctor, feeling as though everything I did or said was being graded. I started thinking I was listening to their lungs incorrectly and that the patient would tell on me—so I'd listen to their lungs longer than usual just to make sure they thought I was actually listening at all.

Making the imposter syndrome even worse, as a doctor in training, you felt you were expected to speak to any specialist without sounding like an idiot, even though they had lifetimes of specialty training that exceeded yours, and to a neurosurgeon, everyone sounded like an idiot. To be fair to neurosurgeons, all the ones I have worked or consulted with are actually kind and caring (despite working days that somehow exceed twenty-four hours) and have been both respectful and excellent teachers.

I did a cursory exam and beyond a sore spine, everything seemed normal with the lad who tried judo chopping fences with his back. So I sent him for X-rays and telephoned his father (a terror-inducing exercise), explaining what had happened and reassuring him that everything appeared normal so far. The neurosurgeon was very nice and informed me that his son had experienced a back problem earlier that year and that I should call him with any questions or issues. I let out a sigh of relief and headed over to see what had happened with Howard and the girl with the potentially ruptured spleen.

The young girl was inconsiderately dropping her blood pressure and Howard was trying to pump fluids into her via the IV. Then I heard the teenage guy calling out for me. I headed back to the trauma room, where the patient informed me that he was losing feeling in his feet. *Why, oh why would you do that?* That was not the type of information I wanted to hear. Suddenly I was alone with this patient who I was convinced would soon be paralyzed due to swelling around his spine and Howard was busy trying to prevent some girl from bleeding to death.

At this point a lady in the waiting room walked back, stomped her foot, and stuck her chin out in a haughty pose, demanding that I examine her sore throat and do a strep test immediately. Ignoring the sore throat victim, I pulled Howard aside and told him the latest complication of the young man having neurological problems with a neurosurgeon dad who I had just befriended by telling him that his son was fine.

I asked Howard if I could give the patient some steroids by IV and send him to the hospital by ambulance. Howard agreed with my plan and I called the hospital to talk with another doctor who, like a true attending, made me feel stupid for forgetting some key part of the neurologic exam and seemed to blame me for the fact that the kid was in our clinic and not at a larger trauma hospital in the first place. He ordered me not to do anything and just get the patient sent to him by ambulance.

Instead, I decided to call the neurosurgeon father again and relayed the updated symptoms. In a lovely moment of vindication, he agreed with my plan to administer steroids in the clinic, discussed the dosage with me and agreed it was best to send his son by ambulance to the hospital. Why couldn't all doctors be so polite and respectful? This guy had every reason to be stressed that his son had a potential spine injury and was in the hands of yours truly, no neurosurgeon, yet he spoke to me as one human being to another. Then Ms. Demandy-pants stomped her foot again and let me know how pissed off she was that I had been dealing with patients who were just lying about in beds while her throat hurt.

In the end everyone was sent away alive and Howard and I sat there again after a long day to take a deep breath and enjoy the beautiful view of the sun setting on the high mountains.

The month came to a close and I returned for my last rotation as a third-year medical student, Psychiatry, where perhaps we could dive into my imposter syndrome.

PSYCHIATRY

I SEE DEAD GUYS

P sychiatry was supposedly the cakewalk rotation of the third year. Medical students regaled each other with stories of their psychology teams being home by lunch and never being called back to the hospital on call nights. It was almost an accepted doctrine that medical students were never called back to the hospital to admit psych cases. Once again I was assigned to the Veterans Hospital for what promised to be a pleasant end to my third year.

On our first morning, we students showed up on time and sat waiting in a conference room. The rest of the psychiatry team ambled in an hour later, shocked we were there so early. "Relax guys, it's the V.A."

None of the medical students, myself included, planned on applying to psychiatry residencies. We all wanted to pass the rotation as painlessly as possible and the psychology team appeared on board with planning an amiable month together.

Enter stage left: obstacle number one to our plan, the super lazy V.A. psychology resident. She had years of experience in looking busy without actually doing anything combined with the seniority to assign us her work.

We learned that psychiatry teams at the other teaching hospitals finished the day's work in the morning, residents and students working together with the shared goal of leaving the hospital to enjoy the spring weather.

Our resident's goal was to sit in her office with the door closed writing personal e-mails. Whenever an attending physician's approaching footsteps echoed down the hallway, she bounded from her lair, rubbing her hands together, complaining that there was so much work to do—even though we students had already completed the work at hand.

The work itself was entertaining. We worked in a lockdown ward and you never quite knew what was going on in the halls or in the patients' heads. There was a range of conditions afflicting our patients: severe depression, post-traumatic stress disorder, schizophrenia and schizoaffective disorder; antisocial personality disorder; and paranoid schizophrenia. The floor was home to a genial sociopath who had murdered people without any apparent remorse, and several paranoid schizophrenics with visual and auditory hallucinations who had killed people based on "God's" recommendation.

As far as we understood, the patients were all properly medicated and relatively safe for us to work with in close quarters. *Relative to what? Juggling scorpions?* Stories did circulate of patients occasionally losing control and trying to break free, requiring all of the team, including the students, to tackle the patient to the ground.

I'm not sure if you've glimpsed a lot of medical students, as they mostly exist in dimly lit hallways; but "tackling skills" is not typically what comes to mind when you look us over. But everyone working with the patients seemed quite relaxed, so we medical students joined in without any real concern for our safety.

As with other medical fields, there were specific questions that were essential to ask in psychiatry. Unlike other medical fields, however, you couldn't believe anyone would give you a serious answer to questions such as, "So, Mr. Harris, are you hearing voices again this morning?"

Remarkably, Mr. Harris answered, "Oh, yes, yes I am."

"And are they telling you to kill anyone Mr. Harris?"

"Oh yes, I'm still supposed to kill the evil ones."

To which I had to inquire, "Just for the record Mr. Harris, am I on the evil list?"

"Oh no, you're fine," he assured me with a smile, "I'll let you know."

You'd think the voices had considered the quandary, that for Mr. Harris to complete his task of ridding the world of evil, he would need to fib, and say that he did not hear the voices anymore in order to escape the lockdown ward. But there seemed to be mostly truthful voices at work in the business of eliminating evil.

That was our rounding duty in the morning; we'd walk around and ask, "Does the television talk to you, Mr. Rodgers?"

"Do you think there are people behind the bushes out to get you?"

And the patients seemed to answer honestly. Except some of the really dangerous patients, they did seem ok with stretching the truth.

We held round table conferences where a patient and several doctors, students, residents, pharmacists, and social workers all gathered to discuss the patient's progress and treatment plan. One morning we sat at the table with Mr. George, a patient suffering from, amongst other things, post-traumatic stress disorder since serving in Vietnam. He had been re-admitted to our service after he stopped taking his prescribed regimen of medications. He was currently taking his meds under surveillance, doing well, and we were discussing letting him go home from the hospital.

One of the last questions was, "So Mr. George, do you still think of hurting yourself?"

To which he replied, "Of course not. I'm Catholic and that would be a mortal sin."

Then the doctor asked, "Do you think you would ever hurt anybody else?"

And again the patient gave a very heartfelt reply that he had been in Vietnam and seen so many terrible things; he could never hurt anybody again.

As we walked out, the attending psychiatrist leaned over to me and whispered, "Yeah, except for the last guys he killed in a bar fight." I guessed that must have happened years ago, but still, Mr. George seemed like a frightening fellow.

The call nights on the psychiatry schedule were, as mentioned, supposedly very relaxed. Recall the unwritten rule: No students were *ever* called in.

My first night on call I went home, got dressed for a bike ride and took my pager just in case. Call officially started at 5 p.m.

At 5:08 p.m. my pager buzzed. I called the psych ward and was told that a patient was being admitted and to please get back to the hospital.

I wanted to reply, *"Are you kidding me? I'm a medical student. Medical students don't get called in for psychiatry admits. Tell the lazy resident to do it."* But instead, I changed clothes, went back to the hospital, and admitted a depressed and suicidal woman.

Depression and suicide. As a medical student, admitting a

patient for depression and suicide was relatively straightforward. Ask them if they'd been feeling depressed, if they'd had any similar episodes beforehand, tried to hurt themselves previously, etc. We needed to ascertain if this was a recurrent problem, something they had been treated for before, what might have triggered this episode, and how to treat it this time. Not that we could do much regarding their responses to any of those questions, but we wrote up the notes and the patients were admitted into the care of a hospital ward that could observe them closely and get them started on a selection of medications to hopefully prevent any future desire to hurt themselves.

We did not have the training to officially care for these patients, but in most cases it seemed like they wanted help, to be heard, more than to end their lives. Fortunately there are more and more ways for people to reach for help these days.

Speaking of which, you can reach someone on a crisis line by texting 741741.

Back to that evening: By the time I returned home from admitting the patient, it was too late for a bike ride and I sat back to watch a movie. As I sat down, my pager rang again, so I called the hospital, assuming I had forgotten a book in the lockdown ward. Instead I was told that I needed to return to the hospital and admit a manic patient.

Apparently there was a conspiracy of black clouds surrounding me, out to make my life more difficult. I knew of no other student that had been called in twice during her or his entire time on the psychiatry team. This was not the record I wanted to set. Then again, no other student had suffered mild amnesia during the first year lectures and perhaps this was karma's way of gifting me additional learning opportunities. So, I went back to the hospital, admitted the patient and was in bed before midnight on a call night, having dreams of shrubbery telling me to admit more patients.

The scary thing on clinical rotations was that you did start to believe you had some of the same symptoms you were treating in your patients. On cardiology I experienced irregular heartbeats; on surgery I was stricken with appendicitis (three times); on pediatrics I thought I had contracted chicken pox; on OB I experienced sympathetic contraction pain and hormone imbalances (thankfully a uterus seemed obligatory or I think I would have believed myself pregnant as well); and on psychiatry, well, there seemed to be a little bipolar, schizophrenic, depressed, paranoid, hallucinating personality disorder in us all.

But we made it through, day by day, waiting for the patients to rush the door and break out into the wild. We were actually taught how to take down patients if they became unruly—which never happened during my rotation. Personally I was quite relieved we never had to subdue a patient—they were all military veterans and trained to kill, while I was trained to measure the size of cervical dilation on a plastic board and could barely wield a tiny scalpel.

My next call night rolled around and since I had already set the record for admitting patients, I figured, with the law of averages, I was free for the night and attempted another bike ride. I returned from my ride, made dinner and settled in to watch the NBA playoffs.

Never do anything you really want to do on call nights; it's a sure way to get paged back to the hospital. I swear, if you stood silently in your kitchen and just stared at the ceiling, you would never get called in. So opening a beer and watching the playoffs was the kiss of death and I deserved everything I got. I was quite excited to watch our very own Utah Jazz in the NBA playoffs. I'm a New Yorker, but after years living in Utah, had found an acceptable duality in cheering for the Jazz, especially during this exciting playoff run.

Tip-off in two minutes...and my pager buzzes.

Grumpily, I drove up to the V.A. hospital and entered the lockdown ward, where I had been told to wait for the patient to arrive. When I entered the ward there was nobody around; the floor was completely empty. All the patients were gathered in the activities room watching the NBA playoffs—just like I wanted to be doing. I figured I had a few moments and joined the hallucinating, bipolar schizophrenics to watch the game.

When the referee repeatedly whistled poor calls against our team (I was biased, not paranoid!), I muttered, perhaps a little heatedly, "That's not a foul, that's a bad call." To which Mr. Harrison started pacing the room, becoming increasingly distressed.

At the same time my outburst inspired a rise from Mr. Robinson, who started shouting at the television, "That's right, bullshit call! BULLSHIT CALL ALL NIGHT! The game's fixed. THE GAME'S FIXED! REF SUCKS!"

A few minutes passed and I made another comment, which sent Mr. Harrison into some really frantic pacing. He started walking in front of the television while grinding his hands together, at which point one of his buddies told him to sit down.

An argument quickly broke out amongst the entire group over whether or not Mr. Harrison should be made to sit down or allowed to pace—all while Mr. Robinson enthusiastically repeated every one of my comments on the game, which I admit to relishing in the moment because it's rare to have almost riotous support of your sub-expert opinions about sports events.

Finally my lazy, emailing, resident phoned the floor asking where I was.

"I'm here on the ward where you told me to be. Where are you?"

"Well, why aren't you admitting the patient?"

"Because there is no patient. There's no staff, there's no nurses. There's me and the cast from *One Flew Over the Cuckoo's Nest* watching basketball. I thought you were going to meet me here?"

I had properly guessed that she was at home watching the game because instead of replying she hung up on me.

Five minutes later the phone rang again. It was an ER nurse calling to tell me that the patient was waiting in the ER and that the resident wanted me to get started. Of course the resident wanted me to get started, she was home enjoying the game.

I wandered downstairs to the ER, which was hauntingly empty except for a nurse who pointed me to the only patient room with a light on.

I looked inside the room and discovered my patient to be none other than the murderous, bar-fighting sociopath, the notorious Mr. George.

I looked over my shoulder and the nurse had disappeared. It was just Mr. George and myself, together and alone.

I sat down and observed my patient. He didn't look too well. His bloodshot eyes kept darting around the room. I slowly realized he was preparing to cut my throat before dashing outside to freedom.

I tried setting a calm tone with an easy going voice, "So, how are you, Mr. George?"

Instead of assaulting me, he confided that he was having a bad night and had started to freak out. In order to protect his family, aware that he was starting to move toward a violent spell, he had checked himself into a motel. Instead of finding solace in the empty motel room however, he started seeing his dead army buddies from Vietnam.

Okay, I thought, *this might be normal behavior for a post-traumatic stress disordered individual with homicidal tendencies who had likely stopped taking his anti-psychotic medications.* Then again I had no actual training in psychiatry. I was merely a confused medical student who wanted to watch basketball.

I tuned back in to Mr. George telling me how awful the drive was from his home. It had taken him four hours to get to the hospital. Since a lot of patients came to our V.A. hospital from neighboring states, four hours did not sound too concerning, but certainly stressful when you thought your dead comrades were riding shotgun.

I decided to continue the friendly conversation and asked where he had come from. He did not reply Montana or Wyoming like I expected, but Redwood Road. Redwood Road was at most a twenty-, maybe thirty-, minute drive from the hospital.

While I pondered how it had possibly taken him four hours to drive several miles, he told me that he remembered stopping at a bar on the way to the hospital—which might account for the missing three hours and forty minutes.

"You know what, doc? I think I might have killed a guy out there."

"What was that?"

"Well, there were these dead guys in the motel room and then I think I killed a guy, outside the bar, but maybe it was my dead buddy. Shit."

Which, at that moment, was the most intelligent response I, too, could muster, *Shit.*

"Doc, we got to go out to my pick-up. There's a dead body in the back of my pickup. I saw it. There's a dead guy in my truck." And he stood up to lead me outside to the parking lot.

Now I'm not the brightest crayon in the box by any means, but there was no way I was walking out into the night with a stressed out, homicidal, sociopath to check his truck for dead guys. Could I reasonably expect his reaction to seeing a dead guy in his truck to be a good one? No, I don't think so.

Would he casually admire the night's handiwork and say, "See, told you. Now let's get back inside. How about some hot chocolate?" No, I don't think that sounds likely at all.

I think I could reasonably expect him to recognize me as the lone witness to his crime, the one person who could put him away again, and decide, *What's one more victim tonight?*

So my answer to his checking on the dead guy in the truck idea was a resolute, "No. How about we just stay here."

He was not easily swayed, but I convinced him to stay in the room another few minutes with brilliant tactical delaying questions, such as, "So... do you *really* think there's a dead guy in your truck?"

I couldn't believe we were sharing this conversation in tones no different than, "So, where do *you* normally go for coffee?" Meanwhile my friends were watching the NBA playoffs and the psychiatry resident was doing anything but her job.

"Well I don't know," he replied, "It's been such a weird day. I swear I killed someone. We got to go out there and check."

As mentioned, I was not falling for the, *Let's go see the dead guy in my truck* routine. This was not the time for me to be playing both doctor and policeman, so when I saw a security guy walking through the otherwise empty ER, I motioned him over.

"Sorry to bother you, there might be a corpse in this guy's truck, could you go check it out?"

I tried saying all that as calmly as I could to not trigger Mr. George's violent spell, but for some reason the guard did seem surprised, "I'm sorry. What did you just say?" As his hand went towards his gun.

"Well this patient thinks there might be a dead guy in his truck and he's not sure if he killed him at a bar or if he's hallucinating. He stopped taking his medications," I explained. "And I don't think I should go out there with him. Could you go and see for us?"

"Where's the truck?" the alarmed guard asked as he radioed for backup to a possible homicide.

"Mr. George, what's your truck look like?" I asked.

"It's a silver Ford, first row out there."

"It's a silver Ford," I repeated for no reason. The guard ran out, leaving us alone again. Mr. George did look a little nervous.

We then started discussing his life, which he told me was falling apart; he felt he had no control. He described his recurrent nightmares and said that the Church would not talk to him; he was not allowed to attend confession. He was convinced he was going to hell for his crimes.

The guards returned and told us there were no dead bodies in the truck.

I thanked the guard and went back to listening to a visibly relieved Mr. George. He recounted graphic stories of his tours in Vietnam, about calling in air support to take out his company's own position when they were being overrun, about having to put his best friend out of his misery when he was dying in his arms. He went on and on and I felt like his confessor to crimes of war. I had long since forgotten the NBA game and could only feel sympathy for this man, sentenced to live in hell after surviving what sounds like hell itself. I gained a small insight into what those men had experienced and continued to live through without much support.

Then again, maybe he was just putting me on like the other day at the round table discussion. I left him sitting alone in the bare room and wrote my admission note and orders.

As I turned to go home the resident finally arrived to the party.

"Sorry, I had stuff going on. Let's get started. Where's the patient?" she asked.

I told her my work was done and I was going home, but she should go hang out with the guy.

"Oh, and there might be a dead guy out in his truck."

FOURTH YEAR: EMERGENCY MEDICINE

A NIGHT IN THE SERENGETI

There's no celebration marking the end of your third year of medical school; you don't get a different colored stethoscope signifying you're superior to third year students, you just move right into your next clinical rotation. There are however two big hurdles at the beginning of the fourth year of medical school. First, passing Part II of your medical board exams. Second, applying to residency programs.

You need to match to a residency program to further your training; otherwise, despite having a medical degree and technically labeled a doctor, you would have no practical idea what you were doing and more importantly, you'd have to start paying off your student loans. That said, skipping residency and finding some tech start-up would likely have been more profitable.

Here is a description of the United States Medical Licensing Examination Step II, in their words: "The USMLE assesses a physician's ability to apply knowledge, concepts, and principles, and to demonstrate fundamental patient-centered skills, that are important in health and disease and that constitute the basis of safe and effective patient care."

Basically, the exam was a comprehensive interrogation of all the rotation and clinical work we had mastered during our third year. Since we had already passed exams on every rotation, why are these tests of our skills even needed? Turns out these scores were screening tools ensuring we were up to par on a national level to continue training, and for competitive residency programs and the medical honors society, to judge us against other students and determine who deserved entry. I sat down two nights before the exam and went through a thin paperback book that claimed to cover all the necessary topics in detail. These board exams were more a reflection of my school's ability to train medical professionals than a test of my skills. If I failed it was because my teachers had not succeeded in their role. Fortunately I passed and magnanimously share the credit for that success with my teachers.

I'm sure that attitude falls under some personality disorder I should have learned on the previous psychiatry rotation; but all joking aside, we benefitted from good teachers (which includes doctors, residents, nurses, other students) both instructing us, setting high-bar examples of good medicine, and forcing us to study all year long; so we were well prepared already; not to mention I harbored zero aspirations (or, *ahem*, chances) of making the honor society or winning the board exams.

The second hurdle, applying to residency programs, was not so straightforward. Applying to a specific program suggested you knew what kind of doctor you wanted to be when you grew into your scrubs. Originally I thought I would be an orthopedic surgeon. It sounded cool. A small problem arose that involved applicants needing to be in the top tier of their medical classes to be considered worthy of applying to orthopedic programs. I was not at the top of my class. My gross anatomy compatriots who never went to class and had wanted to be surgeons since conception, they were at the top of the class.

One helpful orthopedist on the admission committee suggested that I do a year of orthopedic research, thereby displaying a commitment to orthopedics.

An extra year? Are you mad? Why would I spend an extra year in medical training when I wanted to be an actor and a writer? So orthopedics was out for me. Alex, the *Family Feud* champion from our physical exam work in second year, he did a year of research and is now an orthopedic spine surgeon.

My next thought was Emergency Medicine because I liked the schedule: intense shifts and several days off a week to pursue other interests. And yet, they too had a sign outside their entry doors stating only top students need apply.

I decided to start my fourth year on an Emergency Medicine elective rotation. I would work really hard, put in an exemplary showing and earn stellar recommendation letters from the head ER doctors. Unfortunately, all the other medical students who had watched one too many episodes of *ER* decided they, too, needed to be emergency doctors. And they all had the same brilliant idea of impressing the attending physicians that July.

So there I stood in my wrinkled white coat with ring around the collar, wondering if I really wanted to apply for an ER residency. Surrounding me were my eager medical student compatriots in clean white coats, wearing pressed shirts and smiles that seemed to say they had wanted to be ER doctors three lifetimes and forty episodes ago.

Every morning we showed up for lectures on a pertinent ER medicine topic such as meningitis, heart attacks, or snakebites and then spent the day or night working in the ER. The ER essentially serves as the hospital's gatekeeper. Patients are evaluated and determined to be either serious enough to admit to the hospital; treatable in the ER and sent home; or possibly in need of more specialized care, like a psychiatric ward. On this rotation, the medical student's job was to go see a patient, do your best to make an evaluation, and then present the patient and their intriguing case to an ER attending who would decide what to do.

I will recount one night of the ER rotation and save the ER stories of foreign bodies, chainsaw accidents, and heart attacks for the residency months, where I spent much more time in the ER with far more responsibility.

Towards the end of the month I drove up to the hospital for a late evening ER shift. I stared out over the city basking in a deceptively tranquil golden orange sunset. All appeared blissfully quiet. From outside, even the hospital appeared peaceful.

Then I walked into a sweaty jungle. A sweltering and stuffy ER that was reminiscent of scenes from *M.A.S.H.,* complete with helicopter crews running to and fro.

There was no air conditioning due to a power failure and the hospital generator could only be used to keep essential operations running. For some reason hospital lights and ICU respirators had been deemed more important than running the air conditioners to prevent me from sweating through my shirt. Apparently my comfort level did not rival the importance of keeping some guy breathing; a guy who, despite our spending a quarter million dollars to keep him alive for an extra few days so family members could stare at him gurgling unconsciously on a ventilator, was going to die anyway. Of the two of us, I was paying to be there and you think I'd get a vote, or at least a coupon for a free lunch, but no. (If you're uncertain, I am joking about the importance of my comfort being on par with the importance of running ventilators; although not joking about the cost of end of life care for patients that we knew were going to die. Might have to remember that flippantly callous attitude however for some future screenplay dialogue.)

The lack of air conditioning on this brutally hot night corresponded with the absence of any serenity in the ER; it was absolute madness. I squeezed between patients lying on gurneys and being treated in the hallways. Multiple paramedic crews, who would spend the night delivering a continuous stream of patients, were wheeling in three separate trauma victims.

In the middle of this humid and bustling jungle, we welcomed Birdman.

Birdman was a young schizophrenic patient who believed he was some sort of large bird and was flapping his arms while hooting at the top of his lungs, "WHOO-WHOO."

I stared around at the chaos, took a chart, and ducked into the room of the patient I was to examine, a young woman who had supposedly threatened suicide that evening. She sat tearfully staring up at me. I sat down to even our playing field and asked her what was wrong.

"My life sucks. Know what I mean? I don't know what I'm doing, I thought it was going to be different and... I mean, how would you know, you're a doctor, your whole life is great."

"Medical student actually," I corrected her, and thought how wrong she was, that I knew all too well about being uncertain and confused. I watched her continue with the story of her recent breakup with her boyfriend and the subsequent heartache. She was quite pretty when she smiled...kind of sexy, actually. I offered her a tissue to wipe away the tears.

"Thank you," she smiled at me again, "What about you? You

probably knew you wanted to be a doctor your whole life, huh?"

I laughed and confided that I was pretty certain I didn't want to be a doctor at all and pleaded with her not to tell any of my bosses. She laughed and suddenly we were sitting very close to each other, sharing our stories.

While she told me of her dreams, I began to wonder if, hypothetically, it would be possible to get away with getting intimate in one of these rooms—sure, I knew ethically it crossed the line, but she was getting sexier by the minute, I was single, the night was hot... and suddenly she was touching my leg, recounting some funny incident. I gulped and realized something was going to happen here after all.

I looked down at her chart and recalled that she was there after a possible suicide. I couldn't get involved with someone with those issues; I had my own issues and I needed to see other patients, not get kicked out of medical school. Not to mention, I barely *knew* this woman. For all I knew she had been hired by one of my fellow medical students applying to ER residencies in a honeypot trap to seduce and eliminate me as a potential rival for a competitive residency spot. Suddenly I felt very flushed and quickly left the room, handing her chart to an attending.

Good God, the heat and humidity were messing with me.

As I discussed her case, leaving out the sordid details of our almost-tryst, I saw two overdosed teenagers being wheeled into the ER. It looked like a fun case, so I grabbed their charts, relieved to avoid falling victim to my medical schoolmates' hired Mata Hari.

The first overdose victim was a guy who had fallen out of an apartment window. Fortunately for him, a car parked beneath his window cushioned the landing. Unfortunately it was a police car. Perhaps due to an overwhelming sense of gratitude, the patient had been inspired to run back and forth over the car several times. The policeman inside quickly assessed this behavior as abnormal and tackled the guy. The kid's resistance to being removed from the top of the car, however, caused his girlfriend to leave her lines of cocaine and run from the apartment in an effort to help him.

In the ER, the major concern was making sure the guy did not have a closed head injury from the fall. Since he was mentally incapacitated from being on several substances, including cocaine and acid, our doing an exam was not too practical. Instead he was immediately wheeled off for a CT scan of his head.

Meanwhile, I maneuvered around patients on stretchers, listening to Birdman's incessant hooting, *WHOO-WHOO*, and examined the fall victim's equally stoned girlfriend, who had apparently tried tackling the police officer.

She appeared quite subdued. I started with some simple questions to assess her level of alertness, such as, "Can you count to five?"

She turned a blank stare on me, then ran her hand over my chest and counted the buttons on my shirt, touching each one, "One...two...you wear blue," and erupted in laughter as I blushed.

She was kind of cute and her finger was still dangling from my unbuttoned shirt (we had been allowed to dispense with ties due to the Amazonian humidity). I wanted to commend her on getting the color of my shirt correct, it was blue after all, but suddenly, before I could embarrass myself by drooling, a blur rushed by me followed by shouting.

Her drug-inspired, yet still gravitationally-challenged friend had bolted from the CT scanner and was running laps around the ER being chased by radiology technicians and policemen. The excitement of the ensuing chase compelled Birdman to cheer on the half-naked escapee with even louder hooting.

"WHOOO-WHOOO-WHOOO!!!"

Despite avian fan club appreciation, the guy was tackled for a second time that night. And for the second time that night, his girlfriend leapt to his rescue, launching herself off the gurney and yelling at the policemen not to hurt him. The boyfriend smiled up at her from the bottom of the medical scrum and pulled a funny face that made her laugh. I was actually jealous of her obvious concern—I thought we had been having a moment together.

I decided to go talk with my other cute prospect of the night.

Peering into the room with the woman who had attempted or threatened or seen a television show about suicide, I saw her weeping in a chair next to the attending physician who was offering her a box of tissues. I was then shocked to see her hand resting on his upper thigh. *What an ER trollop!* I slunk away, crestfallen.

Later that night the ambulance crew wheeled in an unconscious young man. They had picked him up at a casino where he had won $25,000 at a slot machine. Witnesses say he raised his hands in celebration and fell over. A blood vessel in his brain had ruptured and he had stroked out. He was twenty-five years old and died that night.

At four in the morning a car accident victim's chart was handed to me. She was doing well apart from a whiplash injury and multiple pieces of glass lodged in her body.

It was late, I was tired, and she shrieked every time I injected lidocaine into her wounded areas to numb the skin so I could dig out the deeply-embedded shards of glass before sewing her up.

Then her sultry twenty-four year old daughter strode into the room and smiled at me, her mother's doctor. It was late. Birdman continued to hoot. Paramedics drifted by with patients. The mosquitos' incessant buzz and the malaria floating between us only heightened the moment. I smiled back at the daughter through the sweltering haze, both surrendering to the inevitable direction the night was taking us; we would soon be sharing drinks on the deck overlooking the Serengeti.

I slowed my efforts, grinned at the daughter, and as I surrendered to the passion of the night, proceeded to accidentally poke her mother with the suture needle, invoking some loud yelling.

The daughter smiled at me again and told her mother, "That will teach you to drive without a seatbelt." I decided it might take a few hours to make sure there were no pieces of glass left in this woman.

And eventually I went home, alone, as usual, with my vivid imagination and some sweaty clothes.

I STILL NEEDED TO DECIDE WHICH TYPE OF RESIDENCY PROGRAM I would apply to. I thought back to my time in the mountains working in the Telluride Medical Clinic. Those had been my favorite months of medicine by far and I decided to apply to Family Practice programs with the goal of returning to work in a mountain clinic part-time while making films or at least acting in a community theater group. It was an excellent decision that perfectly matched the lifestyle I desired and I questioned it every step of the way.

Next I had to look at where I would apply. I read a large book with a list of residency programs throughout the country, checking how much overnight call was expected and how much recreational fun I could have in the surrounding town. Realistically I figured I had a good chance of staying where I was and continuing my happy existence.

I wrote yet another essay on *Who I am and why I want to be a Family Practice doctor-* type nonsense, filled in a few thousand dots with a No. 2 pencil, sent away a check with my application, and returned to fourth-year medicine.

SPORTS MEDICINE

HOW NOT TO WIN A SPORTS FELLOWSHIP

Sports medicine, by name alone, sounded exciting— maybe this was my future—a family practice residency followed by a sports fellowship. I could envision being on the sidelines of major sporting events, helping professional athletes recover from injuries, maximizing their potential, and playing a lot of pickup games with them as they prepared for a championship match. I had experienced a Sports Medicine rotation during my third year: After weeks of sleeping in the hospital, performing early morning bowel habit interrogations and stumbling through humbling presentations, it had been a welcome respite to enjoy an "out-patient" elective. "Outpatient" being outside the hospital, i.e. nothing to do with patients living inside the hospital.

The doctor I worked with during my third year had finished not one, but two fellowships. Apparently he had extra time on his hands. He completed his residency (the years of study after medical school), completed a one year Sport's fellowship and then, unsure what to do in real life, decided to do a Rheumatology fellowship. He'd also been the goalie on his college soccer team. He reminded me of these three facts on an hourly basis.

"I'm a sports doctor, that's really what I specialize in."

"Ok."

"I actually completed two fellowships."

"I heard."

"You know, I played goalie for my college soccer team. I'm really into sports. That's why I'm a sports doctor. Did you know that?"

I did know, because he kept reminding me.

But, for as much as he advertised being a sports doctor (which did sound cool), the vast majority of his patients visited with rheumatology problems, i.e. aches and arthritis. Despite the athletic sounding title of sports doctor, which deluded one into believing he was sitting sideline with a major sports team, tending wounded athletes, he actually spent his days writing prescriptions for people wanting pain medication—in between reminding me how sporty he was.

Entire days were spent writing prescriptions for ibuprofen, acetaminophen and prednisone—common drugs whose side effects respectively include: stomach bleeds, liver failure and immune suppression. I waited for a single sports oriented injury to limp through the doors. Instead, the doctor wrote prescription after prescription for methotrexate for patients with rheumatoid arthritis. He told the patients to come back next week to be re-evaluated—great Medicare reimbursements for a five-minute visit—while simultaneously reminding me that he had played collegiate soccer.

By my third day I expected to show up and find him dressed in his college goalie soccer uniform, tossing me a ball to shoot at him.

The only "sports" oriented thing we did was physical exams for high school sport's teams. I enjoyed these exams because they got us out of the office; however, they were also quite stressful. First of all, the players all had to bring in a cup of urine to be tested and I thought I was taking a break from bodily fluids. Secondly, being responsible for clearing these students to participate in sports meant that I was also culpable if I missed some potentially fatal heart defect or murmur. I became convinced that every student I cleared was going to collapse on the field. Despite having spent time on the cardiology service, where apparently I had learned nothing, I decided that every player was a walking cardiac time bomb. I determined it was far safer for all of us if I failed every athlete so they could stay at home reading poetry.

So my third year Sports Medicine rotation, besides allowing me to catch up on sleep, had not provided much sporty inspiration. But I remained optimistic that it was a career worth considering and chose to further explore it now in my fourth year.

I found myself working with a sports doctor who ran the Sports Fellowship program, so it behooved me to impress him. He did unique work: rib adjustments, hip alignments, foot joint manipulations—he took a very holistic, whole-body approach to sports medicine. He had honed his techniques over many years, written papers on the subject, worked with professional athletes, and was considered an expert in his field.

He gave me a ten-minute overview of his life's work, including an explanation of how to evaluate and treat patients using the methods he had perfected over decades and now expected me to use with similar mastery. No problem, right? Just do exactly what he had told me to do.

For the next month he appeared both shocked and disappointed every time I could not properly diagnose a patient using his techniques. I really think he could have stopped acting so surprised every time I proved myself unable to diagnose hip and back alignment issues, because I was wrong every single time. I was, if anything, consistent.

As for sports medicine being "exciting," the first injury I evaluated was a 57-year-old woman who had strained her back mopping the kitchen.

The second part of this rotation entailed me being the sports physician at high school football games. Finally! Attending live games was exactly what I had imagined we would be doing—working the sidelines of sporting events as the team doctors. I had images of exhorting our team at the state championships, their star players overcoming threatening injuries thanks to our care.

According to my mentor, the key to being a good team doctor was to watch the game carefully, that way if anybody got hurt we would have witnessed the mechanism of injury, i.e., the big guy fell onto the little guy's lateral knee causing valgus stress which could damage the Medial Collateral Ligament.

So we observed the game carefully and the doctor would say things such as, "Watch the tight end on the draw... Oh, ouch! I think he tweaked his ankle, inversion injury. What do you think?"

I grew up in England and to this day could not tell you if the tight end was on offense, defense, or locker room banter about the quarterback's mother. I had no idea where to look. I spent that high school football season nodding my head a lot. The team we followed managed to be defeated every game that season; and the only injury I treated at a game was a male cheerleader who strained his wrist catching a girl during some aerial cheerleading maneuver.

My thoughts of being a Sports Doctor were now similarly strained. I had applied to Family Practice residency programs, which allowed me the option of applying to sports fellowships in the future; but I still questioned if general practice was what I wanted to be doing. When I thought of doctors, I pictured gowned surgeons around an operating table; but I wanted a life that included lots of time outside a hospital. All the surgeons I knew actually seemed to enjoy being in the hospital. Still conflicted, it was time for me to start what was known as a Sub-Internship, where I would work as the intern at my local family practice program. If I wanted them to accept me into the program, I would need to display a strong desire, however uncertain, of becoming a family practice doctor.

SUB-INTERNSHIP AND THE
INTERVIEW CIRCUIT

EXCUSE ME, SIR, YOU HAVE TWENTY-ONE

D uring our fourth year we were required to sign up for a sub-internship clinical rotation (sub-I), whereby we essentially worked as Interns. Interns are first-year residents and shoulder the bulk of workload for their team. A sub-I was expected to work at an intern level with a slightly reduced workload.

The majority of students chose to do their sub-I rotation in the field where they were applying to residency; truly ambitious students (i.e. not me) requested a sub-internship at the actual residency program where they hoped to be accepted. This was a chance to shine. If you busted your ass all month, looked like a star and got along well with people in the program, you raised your chances of acceptance. Conversely, if you did a poor job or for some random reason brushed the hair of someone in the program the wrong way, you screwed up any chance of acceptance whatsoever.

I did my sub-I in Family Medicine at the University of Utah where I ended up doing my residency, not because I was ambitious, but because I could not afford to pay to live somewhere else for the month. I will not rehash the same stories you have to look forward to when I go into the details of being an actual resident in the next books. The food never changed, the patients were the same (often literally the same exact patient) and so we can skip this month altogether knowing I must have done a bang-up job.

We were getting close to the month of December, typically the time period that residency programs allotted for interviews. My first interview was scheduled at the same residency program where I was already working as the sub-intern. I wanted to make a good impression so as to match there and not have to pack my bags to leave town.

Despite being in the hospital since 5:30 a.m. the previous morning, I actually managed to be late for the start of my residency interview. Nothing like being tardy to really impress the powers that be.

The overnight resident, a.k.a. the mole, I worked under, had decided I needed to finish a whole mountain of work the morning of the interview, including transferring a patient from the ICU at the last minute right before the interviews were about to start. The resident was either super lazy or purposefully screwing up my chances of being accepted. A normal resident would have said, "You've got an interview that impacts your life, I'll transfer the patient, you go get ready and be on time. Good luck." But no, this resident shrugged and said, "Well, you better hurry up."

Hurry up, that's what every patient dreams is the motivating factor behind their healthcare, right? Not being meticulous, or caring, or thorough, or engaged, but, hurried up. Once again, healthcare at its finest.

Transferring a patient did not mean merely wheeling them

onto the regular hospital floor and waving goodbye as you pushed their hospital bed towards the nursing station. Transferring required a lengthy note about the patient's history and reason for transfer along with all the medical treatment orders: what they could eat, medication regimen, etc.; it was time consuming social work. Knowing I was scheduled for my residency interview and giving me work to make me late was a real jerk move by the resident. Was he trying to make me late on purpose? Yes. Yes he was. Perhaps he had been paid off to sabotage my chances of acceptance.

But I can play that game too. I needed to figure out a counter plan while I scribbled out orders for Mr. Jones' breakfast of IV fluid nutrition.

I figured I could miss the introduction that involved sitting with ten other candidates in suits watching a slide show of residents having a good time in the city where I had already lived for six years. I cunningly figured out how to make the resident's ploy backfire...

I finished my work, cleaned myself up enough to appear presentable yet mildly haggard, and waited until I heard the slide show wrapping up. Then, still wearing my white coat and scrubs, I strolled into the interview conference room of candidates all wearing matching, dull gray suits.

I paused until, with all eyes on me, I apologized: "Sorry I'm late. Some ICU patients I admitted last night needed attention." To be honest, my only real concern was missing out on the lasagna and brownies traditionally served at these events. But my impression was solidified as the guy who prioritized ICU patient care over his residency interview. *Game, set and match, thank you very much.* Everyone else go home now.

The interviews themselves turned out to be a piece of cake as I had already worked with everyone on the selection committee. The committee seemed genuinely interested in my matching with the program and before I could say anything to change their mind, I was paged back to the ICU and told to get back to work without brownies or lasagna.

Once I realized I stood a good chance of being accepted into this residency program, I cancelled most other interviews around the country and kept a select few that were not too far away.

My next residency interview was in Reno and I flew out there after a sleepless sub-intern call night. My plan was to use the flight to catch up on sleep. The people next to me, however, decided to use my naptime to get to know one another better and share family stories about Disneyland. I did not sleep at all and arrived in Reno completely fatigued and despising anything to do with Disney or flying, including birds for no rational reason.

The Reno residency program had reserved rooms for we interviewees at the Circus-Circus hotel, which, like everything else in Reno, had a casino. I boarded the hotel monorail to go to my room and considered going to sleep right away because the residency program had scheduled a van to pick us up at 7:00 a.m.

Did I mention there was a casino?

I would like to say my motivation for hitting a casino the night before a job interview after already being sleep-deprived due to sleepless call nights was based upon a desire to examine the population I might care for should I end up living in Reno the next few years—but that would be lying. The truth was that the thought of tequila and blackjack sounded fun. When in Reno...

When the night started I was already exhausted and broke. By 4:00 a.m. I was falling asleep in between hands at the blackjack table and struggling with simple math problems, like adding eight plus thirteen. Here's something to think about: In that same sleep deprived state that was making me fumble with kindergarten level addition, I was often calculating doses of medicines for cardiac patients in the ICU—albeit without the tequila, I promise.

At one point early in the morning, I folded my hand and the dealer rudely woke me up with, "Excuse me sir, you have 21. Sure you want to fold?" He must have been an excellent dealer as I was up $800 from the original $40 I had left to my name.

I tipped the dealer for his math tutoring, went to bed, and proceeded to miss the 7:00 a.m. van.

I didn't really think anyone would be too prompt in Reno on a cold morning. So I stood curbside at 7:05, figuring the van had not shown up yet. December in Reno is cold by the way. Finally at 7:30, shivering, I figured they had forgotten me and I called for a taxi.

When I arrived at the interview 45 minutes late, all the other interviewees were seated. They had all dressed exactly as the residency book on *How to Win Interviews for Residency* had suggested: nine of the ten women wore scarves to appear professional but have a dash of flair. We must have been confined from the real world for too long if, as adults, mere months from becoming doctors, we had to be told how to dress.

I stumbled into the conference room, hoping not to trip on the carpet, while I honed in on the coffee supply through bloodshot eyes and announced, "Well, this can't look very good."

We were then shown the offices of the staff, which contained a lot of ski photos. The photo viewing quickly segued into a discussion about backcountry skiing and my time guiding skiing in France. Suddenly the hung-over late guy was getting along with the selection committee, and the other interviewees were trying to interrupt with shoddy, kiss-ass questions about the residency- program-associated hospitals and the medical training.

We then went to lunch with the residents—all of whom had been excused from their clinical duties to dine with us in the hospital cafeteria. The lunch situation blew my mind. They had a sit-down dining area with menus and servers—they ate this way every day! A deluxe meal in our program was having a drug rep bring pizza and hand out free pens.

After several minutes of waiting for the sommelier to appear with the wine list, which never happened, I clued back into the conversation at the table where the residents were extolling the fact that they could excuse themselves from the hospital whenever they needed. If they wanted to go see their family, or perhaps needed to ski, they just took off (except for call, obviously). This place was fantastic. I loved it. I could supplement my wages playing blackjack and pay off my massive medical school loans. I could skip work and eat a sit down lunch every day. I would learn absolutely nothing. I must never even consider applying here.

For the rest of the interview day we were shown all sorts of really interesting things, like a ten-foot-tall portrait of some famous pharmacist from Reno. Around the same time that several other candidates were asking questions about this pharmacist's life, my exhaustion set in and I became slaphappy. Staring at a portrait of some famous Reno pharmacist while trying to appear impressed was just about the stupidest thing I could imagine at that point. I started laughing and could not stop until I was put on a plane home.

Showing up 45 minutes late, hung-over, and laughing at the

hospital's prized pharmacist's portrait did not bode well for me being placed high on the program's match list.

I arrived home, thrilled at the prospect of climbing into my bed, only to be reminded by Scott that we had plans to go to his girlfriend's house for dinner. I could barely see straight, but Scott pressed that it was important. Scott and his girlfriend were deservedly concerned about my complete lack of any social life, and had invited a friend over to try and set us up on a blind date. She was stunningly beautiful, intelligent, worked for some huge IT firm, taught aerobic classes in the early morning, and wore a very tight red sweater. *Wow*. I remember thinking she was completely out of my league, just *wow*, and a body to launch a thousand—

—I then proceeded to display my profound interest in her by falling asleep on my friend's kitchen floor and drooling profusely. To be fair, I had not slept in days, and later discovered she had a boyfriend whose marriage proposal she had yet to reply to—apparently my pathetic display did little to hinder their engagement. Such is the life of a medical student.

NEUROLOGY

A CHAPTER TO INSPIRE NO CONFIDENCE

I f you had a rotation that did not fit your medical interests, or that you simply wanted to avoid, then December and January of your fourth year were good months for that rotation because you would be legitimately absent as those months were typically when residency programs scheduled their interviews. My medical school had just increased our Neurology service requirement from two weeks to four—so technically, if I missed two weeks interviewing, I would still be neurologically on par with all the medical students from previous years.

The neurology people however, did not see quite the same positive spin or logic, and forbid all of us from leaving for any interviews. The threat did not seem empty as they qualified it by saying they would fail us, and if we failed, then we could not graduate and proceed with medical training.

This attitude was typical of the medical bureaucracy mindset; we obviously needed to interview to be accepted into a residency program in order to continue our medical training, but were not being allowed to do so. In a show of unity, we students decided to ignore the neurology department's threats. One student, whom I had always considered a pudgy, pasty lad with little to say, forever earned my jealous respect by showing up only three days out of the entire month, claiming he was interviewing the other twenty-eight days.

As it turned out I only had several interviews anyway, having cancelled all those outside driving range and couches to sleep on; my Reno interview blackjack earnings were all I had for rent, food and travel that month.

The days on the Neurology service were pretty easy for medical students. We received an early morning lecture and then proceeded to the neurology clinic where we each evaluated several patients and then left for the day. None of us planned to be neurologists.

Neurology is actually an interesting field of medicine, where the goal involves putting together a puzzling group of symptoms to figure out what's gone wrong with the patient. If a patient has numbness on the left side of his body, cannot feel the difference between hot and cold on his right leg, is unable to see anything in the upper right field of vision, and when he draws a clock, places all the numbers on the right side—then where is the tumor in his brain? I have no idea, but that's the game of neurology.

If that sounds interesting and you want more neurology, then read *The Man Who Mistook his Wife for a Hat*, by neurologist Oliver Sacks.

Sadly the patients we saw were not the complex puzzles that were fun to discuss in lectures or books. Nearly every patient we saw in clinic had suffered a stroke or TIA (Transient ischemic attack, a.k.a. mini-stroke) and we redundantly asked every patient to smile at us, stick their tongue out at us, and to balance with their arms held in front of their bodies while their eyes were closed.

The only catch to this otherwise easy rotation was giving a presentation. I cannot remember what subject I chose to discuss, but I do remember starting to laugh because I could not read the notes I had scribbled to myself the night before. The student next to me then started laughing when he saw how unintelligible my notes were. I started improvising and somehow received a great grade.

But wait, how in the world would I survive as a doctor with that limited knowledge of neurology? Fear not, future patients. In later years as a medical resident (or, spoiler alert, when I become an actual doctor, possibly yours), admitting a patient with confusing neurological symptoms, I had no reason to fret. Why not? My job was not unraveling the neurologic mystery; my job was to page the neurologist on call for an expensive consult.

The neurology doctor then ordered thirty-seven tests and studies, none of which showed anything, but all of which were very pricey. After that, the neurology team would exit with a shoulder shrug, saying they found nothing conclusive, leaving us to care for the patient. I kid you not, every neurology consult we ordered for a patient admitted to the hospital was given a massive battery of high-cost tests, and then the neurology team left a written chart note that the tests were inconclusive.

Have you ever tried to get yourself scheduled to see a neurologist? They have a three-month wait list. Why? Because they're busy ordering expensively inconclusive tests. That's neurology.

ANESTHESIA

A NUMBINGLY STUPID QUESTION

It was now into the last half of my fourth year and I had scheduled the last of my residency interviews for this time period. However, after my initial interview experiences included a hangover, one cafeteria lunch too many, and a sub-conscious inability to arrive on time, I decided I was tired with the whole process and canceled the rest of my interviews.

This might seem rash to those of you who recognize that residency interviews are a step on the path towards a medical career, but Good God, the food was awful, and I had resorted to entertaining myself in the interviews by daydreaming about skiing, friends, my lack of a dating life—anything but medicine. My earlier political studies rescued me when a difficult interview question interrupted my moments of fantasy and I had no idea what had been asked, "Before we talk about that, I have a question about what we were discussing earlier, regarding your program's call schedule." U.S. politics saving me with the fine ability to talk without saying anything.

Instead of more interviews, I chose to sign up for an elective anesthesia rotation. Students worked in the operating rooms learning how to sedate patients with drugs, how to intubate them, and then you talked with the anesthesiologist while the surgery was performed.

Unless you became an anesthesiologist, it was unlikely you would use many of the drugs they used to sedate and paralyze patients undergoing surgery. But they also had to use their skills and medicines to lower or raise blood pressure, heart rates, fluid levels; and there were few, if any, rotations where you would be able to see and, just maybe, practice the scary art of intubation.

Intubating a patient was a procedure that rightfully intimidated medical students and residents. It sounds simple: stick a tube in a patient's mouth and down their airway so that they can breathe. But you had different mouth sizes, so different tubes were needed. Many people had big tongues you needed to move out of the way so you did not shove their tongue down their throat and suffocate the patient. In order to move the tongue out of the way and semi-visualize where the tube was going, you used a laryngoscope, a metal tool that looked like a hand held gaffing hook with a light. The laryngoscope (make sure to pick the right size) shoved the tongue aside, hopefully not breaking any teeth in the process and the intubation tube was passed into the trachea...hopefully; otherwise, the patient requiring intubation to stay alive would instead have a lot of precious air pumped into their stomach; or, if the tube went too far down the trachea, pumped air would over-inflate one lung. So intubation was stressful for doctors in training.

Patients are not too happy being intubated either, as the laryngoscope or intubation device gags them—fortunately they were either sedated or coding and unconscious. During a code situation requiring rapid intubation, you need to get it right quickly in a very stressful environment—not many doctors were going to stand by with a suffocating patient and let a medical student (or resident) try and try again until they get it right. An attending would physically bump a resident out of the way, ripping the laryngoscope out of their hands and quickly intubate the patient. So practicing with an anesthesiologist during the calm start to a surgery, with the patients sedated, with time to make sure the intubation tube is properly placed, was a great way to practice, and become well trained to calmly perform the same procedure during a hectic code situation.

On the first day of anesthesia, I showed up with another medical student and learned there was no real protocol for us to follow. We stood outside the Operating Room suites for forty minutes asking anybody wearing scrubs what we should do. Eventually a busy person involved with anesthesia told us to go find an OR and hang out. So we went and hung out in the OR.

Anesthesia cases, similar to obstetrics cases, were usually very routine, albeit somewhat frightening because the doctor, as mentioned above, controlled the patient's pain, breath, blood pressure, i.e. their life, with all sorts of drugs and machines. And as with OB, when routine went out the window, well, shit hit the fan and these doctors had to maintain calm and peace of mind while scrambling to keep an unconscious patient alive who was cut wide open.

One minute an anesthesiologist was discussing her favorite ski runs or looking over her stock quotations and suddenly an alarm sounded and the surgeon was yelling from inside a patient's belly to get the patient's blood pressure back up— which meant everyone else's was now hyper-elevated. The anesthesiologist would inject medicines, increase rate of IV fluid into the patient, wonder what the hell was going on, and hope the patient did not die. It was quite exciting when a person on the operating room table crashed; but the anesthesiologists were amazing, totally cool under immense pressure. As everything was going bananas around them, machines pinging, surgeons shouting, the patient dying, the anesthesiologists reminded me of test pilots in Tom Wolfe's *The Right Stuff...Plan A not working, let's try Plan B...that's not working either, let's go to Plan C...OK, we're back and flying smoothly... but in this case it was figuring out why the blood pressure was plummeting to near fatal levels...Was the patient bleeding uncontrollably? Increase IV fluids...any change? No? OK, we've got a heart arrhythmia, let's inject something to get back to sinus rhythm...*And so it went until the patient was stable.

While we students just watched the work in the OR, afraid to interfere with anything vital, we did have a pre-surgery assignment. We were supposed to prepare patients to go into surgery. First we interviewed the patients, covering their complete medical history so that any reason the patient might have a heart attack on the operating table would not be overlooked. Then we were supposed to place an IV in the patient's arm.

I had seen nurses place IVs during the past couple years and had placed central lines into patients' necks and groins, but had no real idea how to start an IV in somebody's arm. Turned out you just stepped up and did it. I still feel badly for those first patients, lying scared, nervously contemplating an impending surgery, comforted perhaps by the fact that their lives would be in skilled and practiced hands. Then two obviously incompetent medical students attempted to stick large needles into their veins and cheerfully announced that we'd be present for their surgery as well.

During those weeks of anesthesia I was housesitting for

friends who were nurses. They owned two cats, one of which was on medication for having "fits"—a schizophrenic black cat. Every morning I had to find the cat, drag her out from behind a couch or from under a bed and stick a pill down her throat. Neither one of us pretended to enjoy this arrangement.

The skirmish typically ended with her shredding my arm. Then, to fully express her gratitude, she would hiss viciously and spew white foamy muck all over the carpet. This traumatic morning routine caused me to repeatedly show up late for OR start times.

I started waking up earlier and earlier to get the morning cat chase out of the way so that I could be on time. But the earlier I got up, the harder the cat hid, as though this was a game and I was finally learning the rules. One particular morning I woke early, caught the cat, sustained the close-to-mortal wounds, left the cat foaming, put on my scrubs, and proudly walked outside into an unexpected eighteen inches of fresh snow.

Snow? Not a big deal because I had a four-wheel drive car and my friend's driveway wasn't steep at all. I threw the car in reverse, and listened to my wheels spin on the slippery stuff. The combination of mild incline, slightly bald tires, and wet snow had conspired against me to create a surface so friction-less that physics had never seen its equal. A slippery, but not insurmountable issue, however, because I was early today, and had a snow shovel in my car—albeit, an avalanche snow shovel. For those of you not familiar with these shovels, they are very small with short handles—designed to fit in a backpack. Their brilliant design causes you to throw your back out so you have to go on workman's compensation, thereby freeing up more time to go backcountry skiing.

I dug and dug, got back in the car, gave myself some room,

put the car in reverse, drove a few feet and started slipping again. I repeated the process several more times, each time growing more frustrated because the driveway was not very steep, it appeared flat. Despite my otherwise heroic efforts and planning, I was going to be late yet again. Adding to my growing frustration were the soaked and frozen flimsy scrubs I was wearing, my aching back, and my numb fingers. I tried backing up again, failed, and got out to dig more snow.

Who should then appear? Three healthy looking men. *Awesome*, I thought, *with some help pushing I should get right out.* I shoveled a few more feet quickly as the three strangers approached. They walked right up and stared.

Instead of asking the expected, *"Hey, can we help get you out?"* These guys inquired, "Can we film you?" I was more than slightly put out by now and the fact that these complete dolts (in my eyes) wanted to immortalize my struggle did nothing to improve my mood.

They started filming me shoveling with my mini sand toy shovel and then one especially bright member of the unhelpful trio piped up: "So, uhhh...are you stuck?" And waited for my reply.

I'm not sure what registered on my face—the combination of shock at being asked perhaps the dumbest question conceivable at that precise moment, combined with my mounting ire, left me speechless. I could not get any comeback out fast enough and was only able to shoot them a look that conveyed the variety of insults and sarcasm constipating in my synapses.

Whatever the look was, it must have been interesting, because by the time I walked into the hospital wearing my frozen scrubs, late and with a sore back, multiple people approached me laughing because they had seen me on the local morning news making a furious and confused face at the "Are you stuck?" question. I later received calls that the same shot had aired on the *TODAY* show.

Meanwhile the anesthesiology guys just smiled at my consistent lateness and the scratches on my arm, mistakenly thinking me a wild and crazy fourth-year bachelor.

HOW (NOT) TO FINISH MEDICAL SCHOOL

BACK ON THE GURNEY AGAIN

The last months of medical school, the final days to enjoy life before starting work as an intern, were a bit of a lame duck interlude. Applications to residency programs had been sent out and everyone was waiting for "match day," the day when everyone discovered where they would be living and working for their residency years.

Match Day is supposedly a big deal. The Match refers to the day you are officially matched to a residency program. After all the residency program interviews, students mentally debated which residency programs they favored and sent away a ranked list of their preferred programs. The residency programs did the exact same thing, sending a list ranking their favorite medical students. And to make the process even more exciting, the rank list process is blinded, i.e. nobody on either side knows how high they ranked each other.

The National Residency Matching Program then uses a very high-tech algorithm that creates the optimal match list to make the most students and programs match with their top choices.

Truthfully, after seeing the archaic state of the medical communities computer systems approaching the new century, I was convinced the high-tech system consisted of some waddled grumps in D.C. pulling names out of hats at happy hour. Regardless how it worked, that was that, your medical school received a letter dictating that you were uprooting and moving to Iowa for your residency training.

Many medical schools celebrated the occasion with formal Match Day Ceremonies involving dressing up, pomp and circumstance, and a big party—as though being shipped out to a four-year slave labor camp was reason to be honored. They announced the student's matching program to an audience of the entire school, family members, and lots of applause. It was a wonderful celebration, unless you were the student who did not match, which happened.

If you were arrogant enough to only rank highly competitive programs without a safety, you could be screwed. The program you thought was going to take you decided they really liked the girl wearing the recommended interview scarf that displayed her colorful flair for working long hours, and there, in front of everybody, it was announced that you did not match.

Gulp. What do you do? You scramble.

They did aim to save students the humiliation of not matching by giving schools several days notice if a student did not match. Then you scrambled to call every possible program to see if they had a vacant spot for you. For this reason most students chose to be home at their medical school on match day so that the school staff could help scramble for acceptance somewhere—otherwise your next year was spent with nothing to do but start paying back your student loans until you could reapply to residency programs the following year.

I was back in a remote part of Colorado for match day,

enjoying yet one more elective rotation working at the Telluride Medical Center. I loved my time working in the rural community and match day found me really enjoying the rural atmosphere as I battled with an ancient dial up modem to log onto a computer. With no pomp, nor any celebration, I read that I matched with the University of Utah Family Practice residency program. Then I got back to treating injured patients.

IN THOSE FINAL WEEKS BEFORE GRADUATION, THE SCHOOL SET aside some required teaching they thought would be important for us heading into the intern year. We enjoyed a massive review of pathology. We sat in small groups and debated medical ethics; debates that had no real answers, such as: what do you do with a pediatric patient who would die without a blood transfusion, but whose parents were members of a church that did not allow blood transfusions? Questions to do with turning off a respirator when the family members disagreed with each other about when to cut off life support if advance directives were unclear.

These classes ended around noon and then we were sent outside to play because once residency started, we might not see the sun again for several years.

Looking back over the previous four years, they had flown by. There had been so precious little free time, that you truly enjoyed every free moment to be human and see friends or just catch up on sleep. And here I was close to graduating medical school and it was feeling a bit anti-climactic. So, with two weeks to go before graduating, in order to spice things up, I put myself on the other side of the patient/doctor divide yet again.

Ancient wisdom said there was good learning to be gained

from time in the medical bed. Plato, in his book *The Republic*, stated that doctors should be made up of those individuals who had experienced illness and injury; therefore enjoying an intimate knowledge of the medicine they would practice.

You might recall that several weeks before starting medical school I crashed while mountain biking. That tumble resulted in an enjoyable hospital stay combined with a loss of memory due to a bleed in my brain. Weeks later, the day before medical school started, I crashed the same bike yet again and experienced Second- Impact Syndrome, which further damaged my short-term memory. Well, apparently I really believed in Plato and decided to gain some additional wisdom before completing the medical school cycle.

After sustaining several more injuries mountain biking, I had decided it was a stupid sport and wanted no part of it. Instead I focused on road cycling. Racing road bikes seemed like a much safer alternative with higher speeds and more numerous obstacles like: potholes, other riders, children, dogs, and cars; all there to help keep your attention focused.

One fine Saturday morning, two weeks before graduation, as I peacefully rode through an intersection, an oncoming car suddenly crossed two lanes and turned right at me. I slammed my brakes into a tire-screeching skid. The driver saw me, started screaming, and eventually remembered to also try using her brakes—efforts that were followed by the sound of me denting her bumper.

I imagine it was an exciting accident to witness because just like in the movies, I bounced off the bumper, over the car and into the sky.

Then I fell to earth, hit the road, and my endorphins kicked in.

I jumped up and shook myself off before the pain hit me. I

was mere days away from being declared a doctor, so I quickly put my years of now truly shaken training to use and started assessing myself:

1) Deep wound on lower leg—can handle that, *no big deal.*

2) I can think straight...*maybe? Good enough.*

3) Neck seems to move—*good.*

4) My left shoulder hurts...actually, I can't move it—*not good. Possible dislocation?*

5) Can't focus or hear too well, just a loud irritating noise in my head—*what is that?*

6) Lots of road rash. Lots of pain everywhere—but I can't focus on it because the driver of the car is shouting at me and crying unintelligibly.

Ah, that's the noise in my head.

The woman, more like young girl, was completely hysterical.

Why's she hysterical? I'm the one covered in blood with a shattered bicycle.

I politely asked her to stop shouting as the noise was causing explosions in my head.

But she wouldn't listen to me and kept crying and shouting. I tried focusing on what she was actually saying in-between hysterical wails. My thinking already seemed jumbled and she was telling me about some car accident.

Of course there was an accident. I was there.

She rambled on about crashing her car the night before and asking me, could we just tell the police that her friend, who was also in the car, had been driving today otherwise she would lose her license.

Well I think losing your license might benefit society with that driving record.

But instead I told her, "That's fine, just *please* stop yelling." At that point I didn't care what lies were told as long as she stopped making my head hurt.

Perhaps it was the shock, but I decided I should help this woman because it had seemed like an accident—at least I didn't believe she'd been hired to hit me, but you never know. When the police cars, fire trucks, and ambulances all arrived, I told everybody that I was fine and would just pop over to the hospital by myself.

For some reason the paramedics insisted on checking me out before letting me go—apparently the sight of my torn and blood-soaked clothes, crumpled bicycle, and the fact that I was speaking very loudly, concerned them.

They took me inside the ambulance for an evaluation.

I explained that I was a doctor and knew *exactly* what was going on. "All I need is my leg sewn up and an X-ray of my shoulder," I said. I guess I was convincing because they agreed I could be set free if I signed some papers that I was now in charge of my own care.

Truth be told I was in shock and there's no way they should have let me go.

The guilt-stricken girls dropped the tattered remains of my bicycle and me at my home. The woman who had hit me, the truly awful driver, said that her mother would pay for my medical bills and a new bike. Then they drove off.

For some reason, at that precise moment, every single friend I could think of that lived nearby was unreachable. So I had to drive myself to the emergency room.

However, I could barely use my shoulder to close the car door and with the shock wearing off, I was in a bit of pain. After a few minutes of ineffective creative maneuvering and a recollection of Chuck Yeager in *The Right Stuff* closing the X-1 door with a sawed off broom handle, I improvised the use of my car's ice scraper, and was able to set off on an excruciating journey to the ER. I made it and was immediately subjected to sitting and waiting.

Nobody saw me and sparked the room to attention with an inspirational film line like, "*Quick! One of our own is down!*" No cute nurses ran to me in slow motion with gauze and bags of ice. Instead I sat in pain, observing the doctors and patients.

In medical school, they taught us to speak to patients using simple vocabulary, not techno-mumbo-jumbo. I sat and watched one of the attending ER physicians talking with a young man whose wife had been in a high-speed car accident.

The doctor told this terrified, shaking young man, "She has an aortic dissection and her blood pressure is concerning so the surgery team is working on her right now. She also fractured her clavicle."

She was probably going to die from that dissection and the husband replied, "So she has a broken arm and that's no big deal. She's going to be fine, right?" Just not handled the way we had been taught—but theory and practice were never that close in medicine.

Then I remembered I was supposed to be meeting my pediatric orthopedic surgeon friend for lunch. I decided to alert my friend to the fact that I would likely be held up a few minutes.

I had her paged and asked the hospital desk operator to pass on this message: "John will be late because he's in the ER."

"You're hurt?" the operator questioned.

I thought my bloody body and torn clothing provided a mild clue, but I nodded, and limped back to the ER.

When my friend returned the page and called the front desk, the same observant operator asked her, "Do you know somebody named John?"

"Most of us do," she replied.

When my friend, Dr. Carroll, finally interpreted the front desk woman's message to mean that I was once again boosting my ER frequent flier miles, she drove to the ER to take care of me herself.

As soon as she arrived, I suddenly went from being persona non grata to being a priority patient. X-rays were taken and my leg prepped for suturing. Now I learned a nice lesson: how compassionately pediatric doctors work with patients compared to the rest of the medical field.

When patients are injected with an anesthetic, doctors usually say, "Okay, this is going to be a poke and a burn, just like a bee sting." Then they jam the needle into the patient and wonder why the patient grimaced since they were numbing the pain.

I sat ready for the "bee sting" line, not new to either side of the needle. Dr. Carroll however, instead of using the *it's just a bee sting* hullaballoo while injecting my leg, empathized with my pain.

"I'm sorry, I'm sorry, I know it hurts," she told me repeatedly as she stuck the needle into my exposed bone sheath. And her compassion definitely helped comfort me. She placed some deep sutures and then had to leave to get back to her infant son. So the ER doc came in to finish sewing up the skin on my leg.

He got ready to inject the skin, telling me "Stick and a burn, just like a bee sting," then jabbed the needle into my leg.

"That's one big bee," I grimaced back. There might have been a few more colorful words thrown in.

And there it was, a beautiful bookend and symmetrical character arc: I had started and finished medical school as a patient in the ER—not as the ER doctor I once thought I might be. I limped back to my car covered in gauze with my arm in a sling for my separated shoulder. I was given a prescription for some pain medicine that I had initially declined, but relented when the doctor said, "Later tonight, it might feel like you were hit by a car."

It did, but it was tolerable and more importantly, compared to the accidents I experienced before medical school, the ones resulting in head injuries and memory loss, this time, my head seemed OK—losing all memory of medical school training would have been an expensive little ride.

A quick follow up regarding the young woman that drove into me: When her mother argued about covering my medical bills and paying to replace my bicycle, I discovered that her daughter was too young to even *apply* for a drivers license. My various lawyer friends showed me similar medical court cases where the settlements would have been enough to cover a new fancy bike, the hospital expenses *and* the massive medical school loans I'm still paying off more than twenty years later. I informed the mother (herself a doctor) about these legal settlements, assuring her that I had no desire to go to court. She quickly relented, paid my hospital bills (which did nothing for my aches or shoulder movement) and bought me a shiny new red bicycle.

GRADUATION

Two weeks later was a very special day, the Mayor's Century Ride, an annual 100-mile road bike ride. My first time on a bicycle in two weeks. I was still bruised and definitely out of shape, not to mention I was unsure my separated shoulder wanted to support me for 100 miles. Topping off those nuisances was the fact that I was supposed to be at my medical school graduation ceremony several hours after the ride started.

My cycling friends figured we could start the ride early and arrive at my graduation just in time. No problem, except we arrived late and the ride had already started without us. My friends formed a pace line and tired themselves out riding with me in tow. Everybody pushed themselves so hard that eventually they dropped off one by one, having protected me in their draft to make sure I made it all the way back in time.

Scott and I returned to the finish together. He cracked open a celebratory beer for me, dumped a cooler of ice over my head (my shoulder was killing me by then), got in his car, and drove at high speed to the university. My fatigued legs could barely toddle up the hill to Kingsbury Hall where the ceremony was just starting. Almost as if I planned it, I slid right into my place along the procession line, just as they were walking inside the building.

We paraded into the large venerable hall and sat down to applause. I then fell asleep and don't recall anything about the graduation except walking up to receive a diploma declaring I was a doctor.

I waved to friends and family giving me a standing ovation in the audience, hugged and kissed the administration staff and teachers on the stage, all the heads of the school, and was ushered offstage, with my arm in a sling and still wearing bike clothing under my gown.

And even I will admit having my mom there, all the friends who got me around the bike course and more, friends who flew in from around the country, having everyone there for a big party that night made me feel that perhaps, just like those inebriated med school graduates in The Tombs so many years ago, I had accomplished something worth celebrating... and we did.

And that is the end of medical school.

Yours truly,

Doctor

THE MESSAGE: "WHATEVER YOU CAN DO OR DREAM YOU CAN, BEGIN it; boldness has genius, power and magic in it."(Goethe) I love that quotation for many reasons, and in this case, if you're thinking about applying to medical school, go for it, do it, you've got nothing to lose and everything, everything to gain. And having just read my story, you should have great confidence in your potential.

EPILOGUE

HOW I ALMOST KILL SCOTT

I had several weeks until residency started. So, after auditioning for a television movie (Spoiler alert: I didn't get the part), I traded the evil mountain-bike responsible for my many accidents with a Delta Air Lines pilot for a first class plane ticket to anywhere. I then flew to meet Scott and his girlfriend for some bike riding in Italy. With an open plane ticket and dreaming of lush countryside and beautiful seascapes, I looked forward to my last weeks of freedom.

Things went pretty smoothly—we rode, we ate and drank, we took in the scenery, until a small incident whereby Scott woke with a sore chest one morning after we slept on a beach. I asked if he'd hit the steering wheel of our rented Fiat Punto or if he'd landed hard on the sand while playing Frisbee? But nothing of the sort had happened, so I told him he probably had costochondritis, an inflammation of the muscles between the ribs.

I was, after all, a doctor.

We continued with long road bike rides through Italy and Corsica while sleeping in fields or on beaches. Scott occasionally complained about his chest hurting, but he was still training hard for his amateur bike-racing career and I was still huffing and puffing to keep up with him. So I blamed his pain on the uneven and rocky terrain we had chosen to sleep on to save money. Finally our bike riding and pizza eating tour ended and we headed home.

I enjoyed a first-class seat on the flight (a result of the traded airline ticket), while Scott was having a hell of a time trying to breathe with the masses back in coach class. In fact he looked downright awful, lathered in sweat with a pale pallor.

I told him to take more Tylenol.

Back home he continued to feel not quite right while hiking with his girlfriend, Rachel. The next day we went for a short bike ride and Scott, a much stronger cyclist than myself, had to get off his bike and walk up a hill. At that point I recommended he go to the ER and get an X-ray. Rachel called a few hours later to tell me that one of Scott's lungs was completely collapsed.

So not only did I begin and end medical school in the ER myself, I also managed to start residency in the ER after missing a serious diagnosis.

Let's recap: my first big role as a new doctor was to almost kill my friend by letting him fly with a pneumothorax.

I was supposed to be a doctor taking care of sick patients in a few days and was obviously not prepared to do so. Twelve hours away from starting residency and I had misdiagnosed what could have been a potentially fatal tension pneumothorax on the plane. This glaring illustration of my lack of proper training did little to build my confidence.

I had asked the right questions about trauma and mentally ruled out pneumothorax, but who goes and rides a bicycle for eight hours with only one functioning lung?

I sat with Scott all night in the hospital and tried to study the Advanced Cardiac Life Support (ACLS) exam that I was required to pass the next morning. ACLS teaching included diagnosing and treating patients with a pneumothorax. Great, I was failing already.

EARLY MEDICAL BLUNDERS ASIDE, I LOOKED AHEAD TO WHAT would be a rapid transition from being a medical student in June, to starting work as a doctor in July—an intern, to be exact, but still a doctor.

Recall the joke in medical school: "What do you call the person who graduates last in their medical school class?"

Answer: Doctor.

Well, I did not finish last in the class despite the head trauma research starring myself. I had actually done well in my studies, but that was a matter of having a good attitude, excellent teachers, working hard, and being able to pass tests. I had a nagging concern of inadequacy that, while I did pass those tests, did I really know what I was doing? Could I, on the spot, be expected to remember essential tidbits of information to save a person's life? I doubted it. So the intern year, which most doctors agreed had the single steepest learning curve of your medical training, was going to be one hell of ride for me to play catch-up on.

I was nervous, a bit excited, dreading the start of that workload and ready to get it over with. But for now, for twelve more blissful hours, I was free, relatively, to sit in the hospital with Scott and study for the morning's exam.

Coming SOON: *Playing Doctor (Part II), Intern Year*

NOTES

1. (HOW) SEX CHANGE SURGERY GETS ME INTO MEDICAL SCHOOL

1. To be fair, I did enlist several college students to help me break him out of jail (where we assumed he had been taken). After mistakenly storming a hotel lobby, however, we called it a night and went to eat crepes.

6. CARDIOLOGY

1. My heart was pounding, I was close to hyperventilating and barely heard the words "Scandinavia" and "heart vessels" so I cannot tell you what the real study was called, but I doubt it was called Uff Da, that's a joke for you Scandinavians out there.

ACKNOWLEDGMENTS

I'm grateful for so many people in my life. My amazing wife and kids, thank you for your love. Hoke, constantly reminding me what is important in life. Chris Waddell, always kindling the fire of inspiration. Brad Lewis, exemplifying excellence as a doctor, and encouraging me to write.

My mother, who wishes I had just enjoyed medicine.

My father, who challenges me to be wiser—I'm not.

Thank you Anne Cole Norman for your fine editing eye, work and suggestions. And to Caroline Johnson for your wonderful cover and patience with my inability to choose between various excellent designs.

Thank you to all the teachers, doctors, nurses, pharmacists, fellow residents and students, support team and staff, all the friends I have had the privilege to work with over the last 25 years, thank you for putting up with me.

ABOUT THE AUTHOR

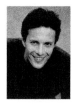

John loves skiing, biking, running, and spending time with his family, friends and dogs. John received his MD at the University of Utah, where he also completed his residency training. He received a BA from Georgetown University where he did not take a single pre-med class.

John has been a river rafting guide, ski race coach, bagel baker, environmental entrepreneur, screenwriter, film director, expedition doctor on Kilimanjaro with his close friend, Olympic Hall of Fame athlete, Chris Waddell.

He attempts to stay healthy, but still falls off his bike (a lot), Fortunately, his wife and kids are there to pick him up.

Playing Doctor (Parts II, III and IV) arriving soon.

Printed in Great Britain
by Amazon

85929272R00140